# CareFully

## 2nd Edition

care professional handbook series

# CareFully

## 2nd Edition

## Lesley Bell

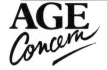

BOOKS

© 1999 Lesley Bell

**Published by Age Concern England**
1268 London Road
London SW16 4ER

First published 1993
Revised 1999

Editor   Marion Peat
Production   Vinnette Marshall
Design and typesetting   GreenGate Publishing Services
Printed and bound in Great Britain by Bell & Bain Ltd, Glasgow

A catalogue record for this book is available from the British Library.

ISBN 0-86242-285-X

**Bulk orders**
Age Concern England is pleased to offer customised editions of all its titles to UK companies, institutions or other organisations wishing to make a bulk purchase. For further information, please contact the Publishing Department at the address above. Tel: 0181-765 7200. Fax: 0181-765 7211. Email: addisom@ace.org.uk.

# CONTENTS

Home in this context does not refer to any form of residential or nursing home care. It refers to people's own homes.

The provision of care to people in their own homes is an area of work that is of vital importance to people receiving care and to their family, friends and neighbours. It enables them to remain in their own homes for as long as possible, by providing support at a crucial point in their lives.

There is no doubt that providing care to people in their own homes can be very rewarding work – and at the same time very demanding. The vast majority of those involved in the provision of home care are extremely committed and dedicated people who frequently undertake tasks that are over and above those they are formally required to do.

Yet the work undertaken by Home Carers (or Home Care Assistants) – like so many other similar areas of work, such as nursing – has been consistently overlooked, undervalued and taken for granted by those in positions of power and authority in particular and by society in general. This is a situation that cannot continue, given the central importance of home care services in the effective implementation of community care policies.

## Who becomes a Home Carer?

The answer is, very ordinary people like you and me! As someone who provides care for people in their own homes, you will have your own reasons for wishing to be involved in this area of work. Many Home Carers have had experience of providing personal care for a relative and bringing up a family. Others have been trained as nurses or nursing auxiliaries. The one feature that all involved in the provision of home care have in common is the desire to work with people and to help them as far as possible and practical.

The vast majority of Home Carers at present are white, middle-aged women. This will change – we need more carers from the wide range of ethnic minority communities who understand the cultural and religious environment in which the person they are caring for has lived and therefore their particular needs and customs.

# INTRODUCTION

The first edition of *CareFully* was published in 1993, since when it has been reprinted twice. There are significant changes in this second edition. This is partly because the NHS and Community Care Act has been in operation now for six years and the implications for practise have become clearer. There is also a need to look forward and consider the future for home care, particularly since the long-awaited publication, at the end of November 1998, of the Social Services White Paper, *Modernising Social Services: Promoting independence; Improving protection; Raising standards*. This document defines the agenda for the future development of the care services in Britain and has particular relevance for the provision of care to people living in their own homes – as will be seen in the following chapters.

When *CareFully* was first published, my Mother lent her copy to friends who received home care. They read it and many commented on the contents. Their ideas and suggestions have been incorporated into this new edition and this has led directly to the writing of the new first chapter – 'Receiving Home Care'.

## The purpose of home care

The White Paper, *Modernising Social Services*, says that social services need to:

'seek to promote people's independence while treating them with dignity and respect at all times.'

That particularly applies to the provision of home care.

### What do we mean by home care?

In the context of this book we mean the provision of personal and practical caring services to people living in their own homes, who for reasons of frailty, old age, disability or illness are unable to look after themselves, without assistance.

# ACKNOWLEDGEMENTS

I would like to thank the many people I have met over the past 20 years who have been involved in the provision of home care and who in various ways have contributed to the second edition of this book.

Special mention must be made of those friends of my Mother, sadly no longer with us, who kindly commented on the first edition in the hope that it would assist me with a second edition. Those comments have been incorporated.

Particular thanks to Julie Edwards then Bedfordshire SSD, Brenda McKie from East Sussex SSD and Brenda Metcalfe from Surrey SSD who provided me with case studies, and to Denise Dewis from Warwickshire SSD Home Care Team for her helpful comments on the manuscript.

Finally I would like to thank all the other people who assisted me with this book in a variety of ways, including, in particular, Peter Dunn from the Department of Health, Lesley Rimmer from UKHCA and David Mellor from the LGMB.

# ABOUT THE AUTHOR

Lesley Bell has led the work of the Joint Initiative for Community Care (JICC) since it began in 1988. In 1991 JICC became a registered charity with a remit to undertake organisation and staff development activities throughout the personal health and social care sector. Prior to that, Lesley led the work of the Local Government Training Board on social services for 12 years, where she was responsible for the introduction of the first national training programme for home helps in 1978.

JICC is currently contracted to the Department of Health to take the lead in the development of the national standards to regulate providers of domiciliary care. Lesley is also undertaking considerable work in developments at the interface between health care and home care.

From 1992–97, Lesley was a Non-Executive Director of the Bedford and Shires Health and Care Community NHS Trust, with a special interest in mental health issues. She has continued her close involvement with home care for more than 20 years and has been Chair of the Joint Advisory Group of Domiciliary Care Associations since it began in 1989 and a Trustee of the British Association of Domiciliary Care Officers (BADCO).

Lesley is the author of *Managing Carefully: A Guide for Home Care Managers* and co-author of *Home Care: The Business of Caring*, both published by Age Concern Books. She is also author of numerous reports and articles on organisation and staff development and speaks regularly at seminars, conferences and workshops on different aspects of personal social care and home care in particular.

A gradual reduction in the percentage of the population available to work, coupled with a decrease in unemployment in many parts of the country – particularly female unemployment – and government policies such as 'Welfare to Work' indicates that we are likely to see an increase in the number of younger people becoming Home Carers and also an increase in the number of male carers.

## How this book can assist

The second edition of *CareFully* has been written as a practical guide, to help you in your work, whether you are a new Home Carer or already have some experience. It provides information, hints and ideas. It is designed to be easy to read and refer to. There are checklists for quick reference and case studies that provide real examples of situations encountered by Home Carers.

This book is designed to help you in your work now, and also to help you prepare for the future by taking account of the changes taking place in community care and in home care.

Some employing organisations may find some of the suggestions and recommendations in this book challenging and difficult to put into practice. However, every effort has been made to reflect what is considered to be good practice in the provision of home care, and all employing organisations should recognise the need to take appropriate action and work towards ensuring the provision of a high quality service.

In providing home care you may be employed by one of any number of different organisations. You may work for one of the many voluntary organisations that are increasingly providing care for people in their own homes or you may work for a local authority social services department (SSD). If you work for a private agency, you may be employed directly by that agency or you may be self-employed and paid directly by the person being cared for, with the agency in the middle, acting as the contractor, introducing you to people who have care needs. Or you may be self-employed and a 'lone-worker', ie not part of a larger agency.

Whatever the exact nature of your employment and employing organisation, this book has been written with you in mind. Similarly your job title; *CareFully* uses the title 'Home Carer' but other job titles are used in practice, including Home Care Assistant, Domiciliary Care Assistant and the original title Home Help. *CareFully* encompasses the work of all who undertake similar activities, irrespective of the actual job title applied or the nature of the employing organisation.

In the Appendices to this book you will find a number of checklists. Appendix 4 is particularly important as it relates to information on formal policies and practices which you should expect to be provided by your employing organisation. You need this information to enable you to do your job properly. If they don't provide this information, ask them for it!

There is also a checklist identifying the components of a quality service (Appendix 6), extracted from each of the chapters of this book. Another checklist brings together all the issues in each chapter of this book that need to be referred to your line manager or some other appropriate person for action or information (Appendix 5).

Each chapter is related to the relevant National Vocational Qualification (NVQ) Level 2 Standards in Care (and SVQ – the Scottish Vocational Qualification).

The information contained in this book will also be of use to others involved in providing home care, in particular people providing care on a voluntary and unpaid basis, either as personal carers, looking after relatives and sometimes friends, often for 24 hours a day, or as volunteers, generally attached to a community organisation such as a local church or a voluntary organisation. *CareFully* should also be of interest and use to nursing auxiliaries and others working for health authorities and trusts, in the community.

This book can also be used as useful reference material for line managers, training officers and employing organisations, to assist in the supervision of staff. It provides basic training as well as reference material.

# Conclusion

No one knows exactly how many people work as Home Carers. There is no accurate information available. The Local Government Management Board annual workforce survey of local authorities identified 75,000 Home Carers in England in 1997. If this figure is extrapolated to include the whole of Britain and the private and voluntary sectors, there must be a total figure of a minimum of 200,000 people and possibly as many as 300,000 providing care services to people living in their own homes. The one thing that is certain is that you are not alone.

There are many other people undertaking the same or similar work as you. _CareFully_ should assist with that work.

# 1 Receiving Home Care

**S/NVQ Level 2: This chapter relates to the mandatory units O1, CL1.**

This chapter introduces you to the range of people who need home care, and their personal or family carers. It considers the provision of care from their perspective and the fundamental importance of communicating effectively.

## The perspective of the person receiving care

Put yourself in the place of an older person who receives home care for the first time. How do you think you would feel? Would you be grateful and relieved or anxious and resentful? These and many other thoughts and fears pass through the minds of people who receive home care.

There are many mixed emotions, which are entirely normal and natural. On one hand people may feel relieved that they are going to be able to stay in their own home rather than enter a residential or nursing home, and grateful that someone is going to come into their home to help them with personal care and practical tasks that they can no longer do entirely for themselves. Many people you will care for, for the first time, will have struggled to cope themselves for a very long time with no assistance and will probably have been frightened about the future. The introduction of a Home Carer reduces both the fear and the physical struggle.

On the other hand, many people are anxious about letting strangers into their house where they will have access to their personal possessions. They may resent your presence, particularly initially and be mourning their loss of independence and hurt and angry that they can no longer do everything for themselves. This is an extremely common reaction and quite natural. As you get to know the person you are caring for, you will help them overcome these feelings.

The husband of a lady suffering from Alzheimer's disease wrote of the sadness of growing apart after 50 years of marriage and the despair this created. He considered that his Home Carer played a major role in reducing the despair and the widespread depression of infirm older people. She was always cheerful and kind and saw the problems of the people she was caring for as something that had to be overcome by working together in a light-hearted way.

 **Do you think this might describe you? Do you think you can work in this way?**

# Modernising social services: convenient, user-centred services

The Government acknowledge the difficulties and dilemmas that can occur at this time and the fact that this is compounded by the complexity of the present system with many different agencies, social services, the health service, housing, benefits agency all responsible for different parts of the care system. They are committed to ensuring that services are 'tailored' to the needs of the individual.

There are a number of new initiatives, including the 'Better Government for Older People' programme which is looking at ways of involving older people in shaping and developing the range of local services they require to meet their needs. Local councils are required to tackle these issues in partnership with the local community.

In *Modernising Social Services*, the Government identifies three ways in which it will encourage services to become more focussed on the needs of people receiving care. These are:

■ Development of a Long-term Care Charter – setting out at national level what people can expect if they need long-term care. The Charter is scheduled to be published in 1999 and its purpose will be to empower people by promoting awareness and making it clear how agencies should respond to their needs. It will also provide local authorities with a tool to set their own standards and a means of monitoring performance.

■ Making services more accessible, for example developing the concept of 'one-stop shops' particularly in relation to joint working between health and social services staff, to avoid people needing care being moved around between different agencies.

■ Providing better information for the general public on how to go about getting social services and requiring local authorities to undertake regular surveys of the views of people receiving care and their personal carers, as part of the monitoring process.

In your work as a Home Carer, you will also be expected to place the needs of the people you are caring for at the centre of your work.

## Paying for the care

Many of the people you care for will be on a limited income, and may be concerned about how they are going to meet the cost of home care. Application to the local authority social services department for assistance will lead to an assessment of care need. This assessment will include a financial assessment of ability to pay a contribution towards the cost of care.

There is currently considerable variation in the charges levied by different local authorities and the contribution people on a limited income are expected to make. All but five or six authorities now levy a charge for home care – either a flat rate or a tiered charge (up to a maximum limit) depending upon the volume of care provided per week. Most authorities do not charge if the person is in receipt of income support, but a part of the attendance allowance is paid to the authority to meet the cost of the care for people who are eligible to receive the allowance. Family carers may resent using the attendance allowance to pay for the care, but that is why the allowance has been given in the first place. Generally the amount paid by the person receiving care depends upon their income and the level and types of benefit they receive. However, there is currently considerable variation between local authorities as to which benefits they will take into account and which they will disregard.

The Government is committed to changing the variation between local authorities for the basis of financial assessment, making the amount people pay towards the care services they receive more equitable between people living in different local authorities. They are seeking ways to ensure that there is:

'greater transparency and fairness in the contribution people are asked to make towards their social care … the Government believes that the scale of variation in the discretionary charging system, including the difference in how income is assessed, is unacceptable.'

The Government will be providing further Guidance on charging policies to reduce the scale of variation. In the meantime, local authorities continue to be able to implement their own approaches to the difficult question of charging for the provision of home care.

One way to enable people to be more in control of the care they receive and therefore more independent is to give them money to purchase their own care. The Direct Payments legislation came into force in 1997 but only applied to adults below the age of 65. In *Modernising Social Services*, the Government make it clear that the age limit will be withdrawn and people aged 65 and over will be eligible to receive Direct Payments to purchase their own care.

# Views of people who receive home care

A survey of 230 people[1] receiving intensive packages of home care found that in the vast majority of cases, people were extremely pleased with the care they received, and were very reluctant to criticise, even in the few cases where there were justifiable reasons for

---

1 Undertaken by the Joint Initiative for Community Care (JICC) in 1996/7– See Appendix 9.

the criticism. This is often interpreted as reluctance on the part of people receiving care to complain, in case the service is taken away from them. This may be true in some cases but the reality is that the quality of care provided to the vast majority of people is of a very high standard and many people receiving care consider they have little, if any, cause to complain.

Criticism is normally reserved for the local authorities rather than the carers themselves, when they reduce the level of service provided or increase the amount that is to be paid for the service.

People receiving care like to have one or two regular Home Carers who they can get to know and with whom they can feel comfortable and establish a relationship. Any criticism of carers is usually reserved for relief or occasional carers, rather than regular carers. However, as care needs become more complex, it is becoming increasingly common for Home Carers to work in teams of four, five or even six. If this is the case, care should be taken to ensure the person receiving care is properly introduced to each and every carer and is given the time to get to know them. It is a good idea to allocate each member of the team as the lead carer or key worker to a different person needing care, responsible for establishing a relationship with the person and taking particular account of their needs. There is more about key working in Chapter 5, 'Making the First Contact'.

In the survey, people were asked what they wanted to talk about with their Home Carer – and whether that was what they actually talked about. Although the majority wanted to hear about what the Home Carer had been doing, they most emphatically did not want to hear about the Home Carer's personal problems. Nor did they want to hear gossip. A high percentage wanted to talk about local and national events.

Few people receiving care wanted to talk about themselves, their problems, worries and concerns on a regular basis. However, a significant percentage did want to talk about these things on an occasional basis – for example when something in particular was worrying them. The skill of the Home Carer lies in recognising these occasions and responding to them appropriately.

## Loneliness and isolation

Loneliness and isolation are major problems for many people needing care, and also for many personal family carers. Helping to overcome loneliness and loss is vital. For many people, you, the Home Carer, will be the only regular visitor. Loneliness may be made worse by a sense of loss – not only of loved ones but also loss of health, loss of a way of life, loss of independence.

Some people are simply wishing away their time. For them, each day is a burden to be borne as best they can. It is important that the work of caring includes the understanding and acceptance of such feelings. They are very real, and time should be allowed for them to be expressed and explored, and for you to try to know and respect each person as an individual.

## Qualities of a Home Carer

What qualities do people look for in their Home Carer? They want them to be:

- kind, caring, cheerful and gentle without being over-familiar or condescending;
- reliable, punctual and dependable;
- trustworthy with integrity and honesty;
- willing and helpful;
- courteous and respectful;
- trained and to know what they are doing;
- committed and interested in the work;
- understanding of the person's needs.

This is a challenging list. Do you think you possess these qualities? If so, you are probably in the right job!

**In summary** People who receive home care are in general very happy with the care they receive. However, it is worth remembering that they will have a range of feelings and emotions about receiving care. As well as relief they may also feel anxious about letting strangers into their home and even resentment at the loss of independence and not being able to look after themselves any longer. These feelings are entirely normal and natural.

# Who needs care?

The number of households receiving home help/care through local authorities was 471,000 in 1997[2]. However, it is also worth remembering that the vast majority of people are able to care for themselves, possibly with the support of relatives and/or friends. They never have a need for a Home Carer, other than perhaps someone paid to undertake household and domestic tasks on a regular basis.

Nevertheless, many people need extra help and support at some stage in their lives. This may be the result of temporary illness, an accident, disability or other difficulty, which means that they require assistance for a short period of time, until they are fully recovered and are able to completely care for themselves again.

Other people may have a continuing, long-term need for care and support. This could be for one or more of the following reasons:

- **Physical disability**, such as frailty, being unable to walk and/or using a wheelchair.
- **Physical illness** which becomes progressively worse, such as Alzheimer's disease (dementia), multiple sclerosis, muscular dystrophy and HIV-related illnesses (see Appendix 7 for explanations of these terms).
- **Sensory impairment**, such as hearing or sight loss.
- **Learning disabilities** (previously commonly referred to as mental handicap).
- **Mental health problems**.

Over 90 per cent of care and support is provided by personal carers – family and friends of the person requiring assistance. Less than 10 per cent is provided by paid Home Carers. However, they are a vital and essential source of assistance to people with care needs who live on their own. Increasingly, Home Carers also provide relief and assistance to family carers in order to support them and enable them to continue to provide care on a long-term basis (see p 10).

We have an ageing population in the United Kingdom. In 1995 more than 10.5 million people, or 18.2 per cent of the population,

---

2 Government Statistical Service, DoH Statistical Bulletin 1998/13.

were over pensionable age. Over 4 million were aged 75 and over and more than 1 million people were aged 85 and over. At the same time there is a falling birthrate so that older people represent a larger percentage of the population than they did 15 and 20 years earlier (Age Concern England have produced a handy 'factcard' including these statistics).

The number of older people in the population is projected to grow fairly slowly throughout the remainder of this decade but to increase more rapidly in the first decade of the next century, with a rise of over 1 million people of pensionable age.

It is very likely that, as a Home Carer, most of the people you will be caring for will be aged 75 and over. However, some people will be 'younger' older people, between the ages of 65 and 74. Still others will be adults aged between 18 and 64 who, because of some form of physical or mental disability or illness, are only able to live in their own homes and care for themselves with the help and support that a Home Carer can provide.

Home Carers also provide care, help and support to families with children. This is generally on a short-term basis as the result of:

- illness;
- family circumstances;
- birth of another child or multiple birth;
- inability to cope – for whatever reason.

As a Home Carer you may provide care to all these people on an individual basis. However, you need to be aware that the needs of different groups of people will vary. The way in which you work with a frail, dependent older person should be very different to the way in which you work with a mother and young child. This is where training becomes very important.

The closure of specialist long-stay hospitals, and the rehousing of people with learning disabilities and people with mental health problems in the community, is leading some organisations providing home care to set up specialist teams of Home Carers who have (or should have) been trained to meet the particular needs of either

mothers and children, adults with physical disabilities, people with learning disabilities or people with mental health problems. In all these cases the Home Carers will be working with the people needing care, providing them with care where necessary and helping them to make the most of their own abilities and be as independent as possible, either individually or living with others in very small groups in their own homes.

It is important not to generalise about people and their care needs, to recognise that each person will have their own individual needs, preferences and wishes, and to respond appropriately to each, according to the needs of the particular situation.

## Caring for people from ethnic minority communities

In 1996, people from ethnic minority communities represented just under 6 per cent of the population. They too are an ageing population. In particular, 17 per cent of the black Caribbean population were aged 55 and over in 1996 and 12 per cent of the Indian population.

The attitude and approach towards the provision of care recommended in this book should apply equally to people of all cultures. However, people from ethnic minority communities have specific needs which may not be met in the most sensitive and appropriate way if they are treated exactly the same as people from white European cultures.

Ideally people from ethnic minority communities should receive care from someone from the same culture and religion. However, this is very rarely possible. If you are asked to provide care to someone from an ethnic minority community, you should never be expected to begin work without first completing an appropriate training course. There is far more you need to learn about cultural diversity and religious beliefs and differences, and about your own attitudes, than could possibly be included in this book. Further information may be found in Chapter 5, 'Making the First Contact'.

Recent reports from the Racial Equality Unit and the Social Services Inspectorate all found that although there were examples of good practice, the specific needs of people from ethnic minority communities were not sufficiently recognised in many places, insufficient account was taken of cultural differences and services provided in an inappropriate way.

 **Think about the people you care for and in particular any from ethnic minority communities. How do you ensure that you take account of their specific needs and cultural differences?**

**In summary** Although the majority of people receiving care in their own homes will be older people, generally aged over 75, home care is also provided to families with children, adults with physical disabilities, people with mental health problems and adults with learning disabilities.

## The role of family carers

Unpaid family carers provide over 90 per cent of personal care, often on a 24-hour basis, 365 days a year. In the survey of 230 people receiving home care mentioned earlier, 50 per cent also had family carers, such as husband, wife, daughter or son. You therefore need to be aware that you will often be working in their home, as well as the home of the person you are caring for. The majority of the carers will be partners so they are also likely to be older people.[3] In these circumstances, the regular provision of a Home Carer to share the tasks and to provide relief can often contribute significantly to supporting the family carer; it will help them to continue to provide the care and so prevent a breakdown in the arrangements that might otherwise lead to admission into residential or hospital care. The reality is that the provision of care for the person in need, however limited, does in turn provide relief and respite care for the family carer.

Home Carers need to recognise the stress and personal pressure that family carers have experienced, often over many years. They will continue to experience these pressures and demands most of the week when the Home Carer is not present.

---

3 Twenty-five per cent of all family carers in the survey were men, 14 per cent husbands and 9 per cent sons.

Pressures include not only the provision of care but also feelings of anxiety and guilt for many reasons, including not wanting or being able to provide all the care for themselves. Fatigue may be common, as a result of demanding caring responsibilities and probably sleepless nights. As we have already mentioned, many family carers are themselves older people and may themselves be frail and vulnerable. If they are not, they soon may become so if they continue to provide care entirely on their own for much longer. Other carers are often also juggling conflicting responsibilities such as child care and/or paid work.

Home Carers should be sympathetic to the situation of family carers. The working relationship should be one of partnership, where Home Carers share the work with and relieve the family carers (for a very small part of the week at least). Take care to not make any judgement about the way family carers have tried to cope in difficult circumstances. Unlike you they are not in a position to close the door on the caring situation and leave it behind them.

The family carers know the person you are caring for, probably better than anyone else. They have acquired skills and expertise in caring for the person and there is much you can learn from them. For example, they have learnt from experience the best way to assist the person to take a bath, visit the toilet or eat their meals. Since in many cases it will also be their home, they will want you to provide the care in the way they would themselves.

The Direct Payments Act 1996 allows local authorities to make payments, following an assessment of their care needs, to adults aged under 65 to enable them to purchase the cost of their care themselves. The age limit is now to be removed and people aged over 65 will be eligible for Direct Payments to purchase their own care. It is anticipated that many of these payments may go to family and friends who were previously providing unpaid care. However, there are restrictions on using the Direct Payment to pay for care provided by partners or other close relatives living in the same home.

The Carers (Recognition and Services) Act 1995 placed a requirement upon local authority social services departments to assess the needs of unpaid family carers, separately from the needs of the person requiring care. This is undertaken wherever possible, but the extent to which social services departments are able to meet these separate needs depends upon the amount of money available for community care. The Government is concerned that in spite of the passing of the Act, key needs of carers may have been overlooked. They therefore intend to develop a National Carers Strategy, the key aims of which include:

■ Empowering carers so that they have more say about the types of services that they and the person they care for need.

■ Considering how best carers who work can be supported so that they can remain in employment.

■ Considering how the health needs of carers can better be met by the NHS and especially primary care groups.

■ Looking to see how communities can better support carers, especially through volunteering.

■ Looking at the specific needs of other groups such as young carers and ethnic minority groups.

The strategy should be published in 1999.

**In summary** Unpaid family carers who you will be working with provide 90 per cent of care. The Carers (Recognition and Services) Act 1995 and the Direct Payments Act 1996 are two important pieces of legislation in relation to the role and responsibilities of Home Carers. A National Strategy for Carers is to be published in 1999.

## The importance of good communication

It is essential that you communicate well with the person you are caring for and their family from the very beginning of the relationship. Providing personal care, at whatever level, is an intimate activity. Somebody else is letting you, a comparative stranger, into their home and into their life.

Establishing good communication can often be quite difficult, particularly if the person you are caring for has some loss of hearing, sight and/or speech or some degree of speech impairment. It can take a while to get used to the fact that a person with poor sight does not respond to you visually, for example by smiling back at you or by making eye contact.

You need to respond with sensitivity and be understanding at all times. You will need to learn when to be sympathetic and when to be firm. For example, people living on their own frequently 'open up' to Home Carers, telling them their fears and anxieties and intimate details of their life. This requires sensitivity. On the other hand, some people are reluctant to do things for themselves if they think the Home Care Assistant can and will do it for them. That is the time to be firm – to encourage them to remain with a degree of independence for as long as possible!

A good starting point at the beginning of the relationship with the person you are caring for and their family is to introduce yourself, saying what name they should call you by and asking them how they would like you to address them.

You should never make assumptions about this, nor call people by their first names unless specifically invited to do so. Many older people and people from some ethnic minority communities do not like anyone other than family or intimate friends calling them by their first name. It is a sign of disrespect to do so.

Good practice in communication includes:

- talking directly to the person face-to-face;
- making eye contact;
- speaking clearly – pronouncing words clearly and not talking too fast;
- using touch appropriately, for example to gain their attention, but not over-familiarly;
- if the person cannot see, or has poor sight, saying who you are immediately upon arrival, explaining what you are doing while you are working and telling the person when you are leaving or entering a room;
- clearly listening to the person, their problems, life history, etc;
- trying to avoid personal mannerisms (eg the use of terms such as 'love', 'pet' or 'dear') before you know for certain that they will not offend.

Poor practice in communication that should always be avoided includes:

- talking too loudly or shouting to make people hear and understand;
- talking too slowly;
- talking 'down' to people as if they are children;
- adopting a superficial approach (eg 'there, there, dear, it will all come out in the wash') or artificial jollity;
- over-correcting the person and unnecessary contradiction;
- showing impatience rather than listening.

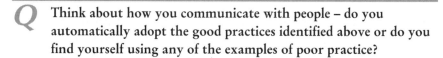

Q **Think about how you communicate with people – do you automatically adopt the good practices identified above or do you find yourself using any of the examples of poor practice?**

**In Summary** You need to ensure that you can communicate effectively with the person you are caring for, in particular if they have any hearing, sight or speech difficulties. Establish from the very beginning the name by which the person you are caring for wishes to be addressed.

## CASE STUDY

**Mrs A** is an 83-year-old Asian woman who has lived with her son and his family since she came to Britain 10 years ago. She speaks Hindi and is vegetarian. Mrs A has a history of illness, diabetes, arthritis, heart problems, problems with voice and throat, fractures and 15 hospital admissions all for different reasons.

Mrs A is socially isolated. Her son and his wife both go out to work. Attempts to provide her with a Home Carer fail because there is no one who speaks the language or understands the culture. Her 17-year-old grandson comes home from school at lunchtime to prepare her food. He clearly resents this.

Mrs A attends a day centre once a week. There is only one other lady there who speaks the same language. Staff at the centre notice that she eats everything they give her hungrily and that there are bruises on her arms and legs. She eventually confides that her grandson beats her up and that she is given very little food.

Attempts are made by social services to get Mrs A into a residential home. Each time she agrees and then is talked out of it by her family. Eventually, after a final admission to hospital, she is sent to a small private nursing home for respite care.

In the nursing home things go from bad to worse. Although vegetarian food is provided, Mrs A can smell the cooking of meat throughout the home and therefore considers the food is unclean. A shrine to Krishna has been set up in her room but she is unable to pray because of the excrement in the home, through the use and disposal of incontinence pads. Also, she is unable to sit on the floor as she is used to in her culture.

Mrs A insists on returning to her son's house, where she is in danger of being abused, rather than stay in the nursing home. A Home Carer is eventually found who speaks Hindi and is familiar with the requirements of the Hindu culture.

## QUESTIONS

1. As a Home Carer, what would be the issues which concern you in this case study?

2. What are the implications for the provision of care in allowing Mrs A the choice of where she lives and the right to take risks?

3. How could Mrs A's religious and cultural needs be better served?

# KEY POINTS

- The Government is concerned to ensure that the needs of the individual and their personal carers are at the forefront of the delivery of care services and that people receiving care are involved and consulted in the development of the care services.
- The Government will introduce Guidance to reduce the inequalities in charging policies and financial assessments between local authorities and to ensure that the basis for charging is both transparent and fair.
- The age limit of 65 for Direct Payments will be withdrawn and people aged over 65 will be eligible to receive the payment to purchase their own care.
- It is natural for the person receiving care to have mixed emotions – relief that they are able to stay in their own home but hurt and anger that they have lost their independence.
- Many older people become depressed with the situation they find themselves in. They look to you, the Home Carer, to be cheerful and reassuring.
- People like their Home Carers to talk to them, particularly about what they are doing and current affairs.
- There will be occasions when the person receiving care wants to talk about personal problems and difficulties. You need to be sensitive and recognise when these situations arise and respond appropriately.
- Although most home care is provided to older people, it is also provided to families with children, adults with physical disabilities, people with mental health problems and adults with learning disabilities.
- Ninety per cent of care is provided by unpaid personal carers. Increasingly you may find yourself working with members of the family to provide the care.
- A National Strategy for Carers is to be published in 1999.
- You should never provide care for people from ethnic minority communities without receiving the appropriate training.
- People from ethnic minority communities should never be treated as 'honorary whites' – that is insulting and patronising.
- Effective communication is a key skill in the provision of care.

# 2   The Importance of Core Values

S/NVQ Level 2: This chapter relates to the mandatory units O1, CL1 CU1 and Z1.

This chapter considers the value base, which should underpin the provision of all home care, and how this can or should be translated into practice. It looks at the particular issues involved in allowing people to make choices and to take risks.

## What do we mean by core values?

Core values are the basic principles of good practice upon which the provision of all care for vulnerable people who need help should be based. They are so important in the provision of home care that if you have difficulty in sharing or accepting these core values, maybe you should think again about the work you are doing and your attitude to the people you are caring for.

There are many versions of core values within the care sector and they come in a variety of styles and packages. Sometimes they are incorporated into a 'mission' statement. However, whatever the core values are called, you will find that most of them have much in common.

You will find that there are two elements to the core values, as illustrated in the diagram on the following page.

On the one hand, there are the **principles** which should underpin the provision of all home care services. On the other hand, there are the **rights** of each person who receives care.

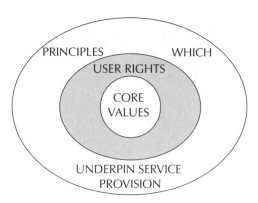

PRINCIPLES — WHICH
USER RIGHTS
CORE
VALUES
UNDERPIN SERVICE
PROVISION

## The importance of core values

You will find that many people use the terms 'values', 'principles' and 'rights' as if they are totally interchangeable. This is not always the case and there are significant differences between **principles** which relate to practice – the way in which you do your work, and **rights** which relate to individuals.

Upholding core values means that you should **implement the underpinning principles** throughout your practice and **respect the rights of users**. Many of the problems which occur in home care arise because Home Carers fail to observe and put the core values into practice. Admittedly it is not easy, but it is essential if this is the work you are going to do.

Most of the underpinning principles are the same, or similar, but put into the context of the particular needs of different groups of people who need care, or the type of care provided.

 Obtain copies of core value statements which apply within your organisation. There may be statements for the organisation as a whole and/or for your particular service. What about your local community health trust – how does their statement of core values or underpinning principles compare to yours?

**In summary** You need to implement the underpinning principles into your daily work and protect and uphold the rights of the people you are caring for.

# Underpinning principles

If you are familiar with the National or Scottish Vocational Qualification and the awards in care, you will be familiar with the concept of underpinning principles, identified in the 'O' unit (or value base) which underpins all the performance standards in care. If you are not familiar with them, please refer to Appendix 2.

The S/NVQ in care is unique among S/NVQs in incorporating an underpinning value base into the qualification. The care standards were revised in 1997. At S/NVQ Level 2 – the level of qualification for the majority of Home Carers – there is one O unit which has three elements.

### UNIT O1 - Foster people's equality, diversity and rights

O1.1    Foster people's rights and responsibilities
O1.2    Foster equality and diversity of people
O1.3    Maintain the confidentiality of information

Competence in all three elements must be demonstrated throughout your work in order to meet the standards specified. The introduction to the core unit states:

'This unit is about acknowledging the equality and diversity of people and their rights and responsibilities. Due to the often sensitive nature of the information about people with which the sector deals, the maintenance of confidentiality is also included. Whilst it is recognised that workers are not always in a position to change and influence structures directly, they are expected to be proactive against discrimination.

'The standards recognise that to acknowledge people's equality, diversity and rights, the worker has to be able to handle a number of competing tensions: within people themselves and between different people. Discrimination against people may occur for a wide range of reasons such as: differing abilities, age, class, caste, creed, culture, gender, health status, relationship status, mental health, offending background, place of origin, political beliefs, race, responsibility for dependants, religion, sexuality.

'The term "people" is used broadly to cover individuals, families, groups, communities and organisations. The people may be clients, colleagues or anyone else with whom the worker comes into contact.'

(Source: Care Sector Consortium)

These principles should apply to each and every one of us, regardless of whether we have a particular need for personal care.

 Think about what this means in practice. Make a list of the ways in which you think the people you care for may be discriminated against and why. What do you think you can do to reduce the effect of discrimination?

How well do you think that you incorporate these underpinning principles into your daily work? In what ways could you improve your practice? For example:

- Do you do everything you can to maintain the confidentiality of information?
- How much do you talk to your colleagues about the people you care for?
- What do you say and share with your colleagues about the personality, views or lifestyle of the people you are caring for?
- If the position was reversed and you were receiving care, would you like the same things said about you to strangers?

## Codes of conduct and practice

The long-awaited General Social Care Council (GSCC) is at last to be established. It will be an independent statutory body charged with the duty to secure the interests and welfare of people receiving care by raising the quality of services and improving performance and by regulating individual people who provide social care. It is comparable to similar, well established bodies in the health service.

One of the functions of the GSCC will be to develop codes of conduct and practice for the whole workforce – including home care. The proposal is that individuals will be personally responsible and accountable for their own standard of conduct and practice based upon the codes.

Home Carers whose personal conduct falls short of that which is required by the code may find their employment terminated.

---

 **What do you think should go into a Code of Conduct and Practice for Home Carers? Which areas of practice should it cover? There are a number of pointers in this book. You could, with colleagues, develop your own code in advance of that produced by the General Social Care Council. The Code for the majority of Home Carers is unlikely to be developed much before 2001 at the very earliest, and probably later, since the first priority for the GSCC will be people who work with children and families.**

---

**In summary** The O unit of the S/NVQ in care identifies standards which should underpin your practice. The details of the O unit may be found in Appendix 2. The General Social Care Council will be producing Codes of Conduct and Practice for the whole workforce including, in time, home care. The Codes will make individuals responsible and accountable for their own personal conduct and practice in work and will be legally enforceable in employment law.

## The rights of people receiving care

As a Home Carer you have a responsibility to the people you are caring for, to recognise and protect their rights. Together, the **principles** identified in the S/NVQ O unit and the **rights** spelt out below provide the core **values**, which should be the basis of all the care you provide to people living in their own homes.

The **rights** of each individual person include:

- The right to **privacy** and **confidentiality**.
- The right to be **listened to** and to have wishes and opinions considered.
- The right to **respect** and not to be demeaned (ie literally, to lower in dignity).
- The right to have **freedom of movement** and of not being restricted by, for example, being kept in a locked room or home.
- The right to be allowed to **take risks**.

- The right **not to be discriminated against** for any reason; for example, race, age, religion, colour, disability, sexual orientation, physical and financial circumstances.
- The right to **personal choice**, according to individual preferences whenever and wherever possible.
- The right to be **addressed** in the way each individual person chooses and prefers, and to have one's personal first name used only on freely given consent.
- The right to have access to preferred **religious leaders**.
- The right to **eat and drink** according to own preferences, only being advised by appropriate people on the advantages and dangers of certain foods and of the dangers of excessive smoking and alcohol consumption.
- The right to **make one's own decisions** – which may conflict with others, for example professionals and/or with the family view.
- The right to have **access to friends** and **relatives** and to be given assistance to see them, if necessary.
- The right to **have a pet** if able to care for and look after it.
- The right **not to be coerced** to participate in activities against one's wishes and desires (eg singing, playing games).
- The right to say **no**!

 Think about what each of these 'rights' means to you personally. Some of them may be more important to you than others. How would you feel if any of these personal rights were ignored? The people you are caring for probably feel the same way.

This list of rights is not comprehensive. Can you think of any others that you would add?

Think about how you observe these rights in practice in your work. Do you think that you show respect to the people you are caring for? Could you show greater respect in any way?

The organisation for which you work may have its own list of principles, values for service delivery or rights. Obtain a copy and compare it to the lists above. Identify the similarities and the differences.

If your organisation does not have such a list, do you think it should have one? These lists could provide a starting point.

People's rights have recently received a lot of attention with the publishing of 'charters' informing people about their rights. Two examples of these produced by the Government are the Citizen's Charter and the Patient's Charter.

## Protecting people's rights and enabling personal choice

Many of these rights are very difficult to protect in practice. It is the right of the individual being cared for to be listened to, to have their views respected and to have their wishes and opinions taken into consideration. This is of great importance. However, the individual's wishes can, on occasion, conflict with the 'professional' opinion about what is actually in their best interest.

The need to safeguard confidentiality is essential, yet you may be given information by the person you are caring for that makes you concerned for their continued health or safety, and makes it necessary to pass on the information to their GP or your line manager. In these circumstances, always seek permission from the person you are caring for to tell others. Never pass information on to others, including relatives and friends of the person receiving care, without that person's permission.

 How much do you tell your colleagues about what has happened with individual people you care for? Do you think this breaches their confidentiality and rights? Would you like the same or similar things about you talked about, behind your back, with people you don't know? No, of course you would not, so it shouldn't happen in relation to the people you care for and their family carers. This will almost certainly be a topic that will be covered in the individual Code of Conduct and Practice referred to earlier to be drawn up by the General Social Care Council.

Someone who has poor sight may prefer private correspondence to be read to them by a Home Carer, rather than by a member of the family, knowing that confidentiality will be observed and that no comment will be made on the content.

On occasions a person who is suffering from Alzheimer's disease, and is therefore confused, may wander around, outside the home, at night, often in an undressed state. The obvious and least drastic remedy is to lock them in the home, but that takes away their personal right to freedom of movement.

Another example is the right to make one's own decisions. This can be a difficult area, which can lead to disagreement, particularly when the decision of the individual person conflicts with the wishes of the relatives. However, the only limitation on this right should be where the medically diagnosed mental condition of the person indicates that she or he is not capable of self-determination (see Chapter 11, pp 182–184).

 It is a good test for you as a Home Carer to place yourself in the position of the person you are caring for, read through the list of rights again and ask yourself how important these rights are to you. How would you feel if they were taken away or ignored? Ask yourself, 'How would I react?' Think about your practice. Do you think you do anything which may take away the person's rights and reduce their independence?

Most older people say that they feel the same inside as they did when they were younger. If they feel the same, why should they be treated any differently? How do you feel? Do you feel the same as you did 20 years ago? Would you expect to be treated any differently?

You, as a Home Carer, should **always** treat all the people you are caring for in exactly the same way as you would wish to be treated yourself.

As the Home Carer you can be caught in the middle. For example:

1 A person with bronchitis and emphysema who has smoked for 60 years might be encouraged to stop smoking (the professional view). The person may reject such advice and their decision must be respected.

2 An older person may become forgetful, but yet insist on carrying out cooking and other activities in which there is a significant element of risk that they may harm themselves. A compromise may be possible with high-risk activities being undertaken under supervision by the Home Carer.

3 A person may be substantially overweight, with the resulting problems of mobility and weight-related diseases. The professional view might seek to impose diet and exercise. The individual may prefer to continue as they are. Persuasion may be tried and might be at least partially effective with some people. If not, the views and wishes of the individual concerned must prevail.

In general:

- Respect the right of the individual to **choose**.
- Try to change behaviour that could possibly be harmful and/or dangerous, by the use of **reasoning** and **persuasion**.
- Seek to achieve an acceptable **balance** between the professional view and wishes and those of the person concerned. This may not be easy!
- Wherever possible, seek to encourage, stimulate and maintain the **independence** of the person needing care.
- **Don't** encourage unnecessary or premature dependence. Remember the right to take **risks**. Few people want to be wrapped in cotton wool.
- Keep the person's family and friends informed of what you are trying to do and why. **Involve** and **consult** them whenever possible and appropriate.

**In summary** Everybody has certain personal rights which you should uphold in your practice. However, there will be times when this conflicts with safeguarding the health and safety of the people you are caring for.

Mrs B began to make a series of formal complaints to the local authority concerning the attitude and approach of her Home Carers. Eventually an official investigation was undertaken.

The investigation revealed that Mrs B's situation was common knowledge among the home care team and that issues of confidentiality were ignored. The general view was that Mrs B was 'putting it on' to seek attention and did not 'deserve' to be provided with home care. There was general resentment against her.

The practice of holding group supervision sessions encouraged the sharing of confidential information and the forming of views about customers on the basis of hearsay and gossip. Case notes, which provided details of the seriousness of Mrs B's condition and situation, were held by the care management team and were not available to the manager of the home care team.

One of the many outcomes from the investigation was that the home care team were given training in the 'O' unit, underpinning value base.

# QUESTIONS

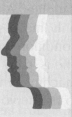

1. If you were the Home Carer for Mrs B, what steps could you have taken to ensure confidentiality of information?

2. What are the significant differences between Mrs B and most of your older customers? How would this affect the care you would give?

3. What lessons does this case study hold for the labelling and stereotyping of people?

4. How can you avoid this situation arising within supervision?

# KEY POINTS

- The core values reflect the underpinning principles of practice and the rights of the people receiving care.
- If you do not accept and share the core values, then caring work may not be the right occupation for you as you will not be able to meet the professional standard required.
- The O1 unit of the S/NVQ in Care identifies standards which should underpin all your work.
- The General Social Care Council will bring in individual Codes of Conduct and Practice, which will make all staff responsible and accountable for their own conduct.
- Many of the 'rights' we all take for granted are very difficult to safeguard in practice. There will be times when you will be balancing the rights of the people you are caring for with the wishes of their family and other professionals.
- Maintaining confidentiality is a key value underpinning your practice and should be safeguarded at all times, particularly in discussions with your colleagues.
- You should **always** treat the people you are caring for in exactly the same way as you would wish to be treated yourself.
- There is an acute shortage of Home Carers from ethnic minority communities willing and able to meet the care needs of people from those communities.
- You should never be asked to provide care to people from ethnic minority communities before you have received the appropriate training.

# 3 Providing a Service for the New Millennium

**S/NVQ Level 2:** This chapter relates to the mandatory units O1, CL1; Option Group A units CU5, W2, W3.

This chapter considers the way in which home care has changed and evolved over the years. In particular it considers the impact of the NHS and Community Care Act 1990 on the development of home care services and the implications of the 1998 White Paper on *Modernising Social Services* for the home care services of the future. It also considers the training required to enable Home Carers to respond to the increasing demands of the work.

## The origins of the home care service

The home care service of the 1990s has evolved from a service that was originally set up to provide help and support to mothers with children and young babies. The first recorded service was in 1897 provided by the Jewish Sickroom Society. Then between the two world wars, large cities such as Liverpool, Glasgow and Birmingham set up their own services.

The modern home care service has its origins in the Beveridge Report (1942) and the 1948 National Health and National Assistance Act, which placed responsibility upon local authorities to provide a 'home help' service, as it was then called. The next major milestone for home care was the National Health Service and Community Care Act 1990 which was implemented in April 1993 and stimulated the next stage of development for home care, which will take it into the new millennium.

Two major shifts occurred in the home care service between the 1948 Act and the 1990 Act:

1 The emphasis moved from the provision of support and assistance to mothers with children to the provision of help to older, frail and vulnerable people who were unable to look after themselves without such support.

2 The nature of the work shifted from a focus on the provision of practical care such as cleaning, shopping and cooking, to an emphasis on the provision of more personal care such as helping people get up from bed, washed, bathed, dressed and going to the toilet.

Both these trends have been accelerated by the implementation of the NHS and Community Care Act.

**In summary** The modern home care service owes its origins to the National Health and National Assistance Act 1948.

# The National Health Service and Community Care Act 1990

The NHS and Community Care Act 1990 introduced new requirements for community care, phased in from April 1993. These requirements placed home care at the heart of the provision of effective community care.

Before the implementation of the Act, anyone who wanted to enter a private residential home, but could not meet the cost of the fees themselves, was funded by the Department of Social Security. There was no assessment of the real need for residential care. As a result, central government expenditure on private residential care soared unchecked between 1978 and 1990. There was no limit on the total annual expenditure.

The NHS and Community Care Act makes local authority social services departments responsible, for the first time, for assessing the care needs of everybody who is unable to pay the full cost of their care themselves, including those who prior to the Act would have

gone straight into residential care. Social services departments are now responsible for buying services from a wide range of providers of care services (including their own in-house services) in order to meet the care needs that have been identified. Additional, but limited, money was provided by central government over the six years, 1993–99 to meet the additional care costs incurred.

People who have the financial resources to meet the cost of the care themselves do not need to have their needs assessed by social services and the department will not be involved in contracting for their care. If you work for a private or voluntary sector organisation, you may well have a number of 'private' customers who meet the cost of their care entirely themselves.

Since given the choice, the vast majority of people want to stay in their own homes for as long as possible. One of the major outcomes of the NHS and Community Care Act has been a shift in emphasis towards supporting people in their own homes rather than placing them in residential care.

The Government, in the White Paper, *Caring for People – Community care in the next decade and beyond* (1989), identified six key objectives for community care:

- To promote the development of domiciliary, day and respite services to enable people to live in their own homes wherever feasible and sensible.
- To ensure that service providers make practical support for carers a high priority.
- To make assessment of need and good care management the basis of high-quality care.
- To promote the development of a flourishing independent sector alongside good-quality public services.
- To clarify the responsibilities of agencies and to make it easier to hold them to account for their performance.
- To secure better value for taxpayers' money by introducing a new funding structure for social care.

These six objectives are now generally recognised as indicators of good and effective practice. The provision of home care, as the principal service responsible for providing care and supporting people in their own homes, was and will continue to be the cornerstone of community care and essential to the achievement of the above objectives.

**In summary** Since April 1993 local authority social services departments have been responsible for assessing the care needs of those people who are unable to meet the full cost themselves. This has placed the emphasis on the provision of home care rather than residential care.

## The home care service in the late 1990s

The home care service is still in the process of change. The two trends identified at the beginning of this chapter have continued, and indeed have accelerated. New trends have also emerged, specifically:

1 The development of the 'mixed economy' of home care provision. An increasing number of voluntary and private sector organisations providing home care, and a corresponding reduction in the level of provision of local authority 'in-house' home care services.

2 Demand exceeding the resources available. A considerable increase in the number of people referred to social services departments to have their care needs assessed, leading to:

- tightening of the criteria which decide who is eligible for the services;
- prioritising the need for care services;
- rationing the provision of care and the allocation of resources.

3 A move towards providing a flexible home care service 24 hours a day, 7 days a week in order to respond to and meet the complex needs of people who are now cared for in their own homes in preference to residential care.

## The development of the 'mixed economy' of home care provision

Up until the late 1970s local authority social services departments and voluntary organisations provided the vast majority of care services. The Conservative Government started development of the 'mixed economy' of care provision in the late 1970s when they encouraged the private sector to move into the provision of residential care. They continued to support the expansion of residential care throughout the 1980s until, by the late 1980s, the majority of residential care places was, and continues to be, provided by the private sector.

The provision of home care services was relatively unaffected until the implementation of the NHS and Community Care Act in April 1993. One of the conditions imposed by the Government on local authorities in England (but not in the rest of the country) was that 80 per cent of the money transferred to social services departments to implement the requirements of the Act should be spent in the 'independent' sector. This meant primarily private and voluntary organisations, although it also included NHS Trusts.

Prior to 1993 there were few private and voluntary organisations providing personal care for people in their own homes, apart from the registered nursing agencies. There were of course many agencies privately providing a domestic cleaning service, but not the kind of personal care we associate with home care.

By 1998 there are known to be at least 3,000 organisations – most of them being members of the United Kingdom Home Care Association (UKHCA). No accurate figures are available because, at the time of writing, there is no regulation of home care agencies, comparable to that for residential care, so home care agencies do not have to be registered with any central body. Anyone is currently at liberty to set up a home care agency if they wish. However, the Government intends to introduce legislation and regulation for home care should be on the statute book early in the new century (see p 42).

A number of long-established voluntary organisations and housing associations have moved into home care provision for the first time, including Age Concern, British Red Cross and Anchor Housing. Other voluntary organisations such as the Leonard Cheshire Foundation have built up their home care provision rather than their residential provision, specialising in particular in care for adults with disabilities.

Many residential homes, nursing homes and private hospitals have also diversified into providing home care, often on a localised basis.

In contrast to the expansion in the provision of home care by agencies in the private and voluntary sector, there has been contraction in the volume of home care provided by local authorities' own in-house services. Local authorities directly provided around 56 per cent of total contact hours in 1997 compared with 64 per cent the previous year and over 95 per cent in 1992[4] before the implementation of the NHS and Community Care Act. Most in-house provision is now targeted on the provision of care to people with the most complex and personal care needs, while more simple and/or practical care support is commissioned from agencies in the private and voluntary sector. At present there are wide variations from the one or two authorities which no longer provide an in-house home care service themselves, at one end of the spectrum, through to those which have retained the majority of service provision in-house and contract out less than 10 per cent at the other end.

However, pressure on the limited financial resources, the search for 'best value' in service provision and the continuous quest to provide more services with less resources, will inevitably continue the shift of emphasis in the provision of home care away from local authority social services departments to agencies in the voluntary and private sectors.

---

4 Government Statistical Service DoH Statistical Bulletin 1998/13.

## *Increase in demand for home care*

Expenditure on home care by local authority social services depart-ments in England in 1995 was a total of £1,028.1 million.[5] Laing and Buisson estimated the figure in the UK to be £1,265 million in 1997. That represents a very large business indeed.

Local authorities purchased over 2.6 million hours of home help or home care in 1997.[6] This is over a 50 per cent increase between 1992 (prior to the implementation of the NHS and Community Care Act) and 1997, in the number of hours of home care purchased by social services departments from organisations in the private and voluntary sector, as well as their own in-house services.

All of the increase has been in the purchase of home care services from private and voluntary sector organisations. The volume of home care provided by local authority in-house services showed a 6 per cent drop in 1997 on the previous year's figure. It is now below the level that it was in 1992.

The increase in the demand for services will continue into the next century. Official figures tell the story:[7]

NUMBER OF OLDER PEOPLE IN THE UK

|          | Aged 65+ (millions) | Aged 80+ (millions) |
|----------|---------------------|---------------------|
| 1971     | 7.38                | 1.29                |
| 1981     | 8.46                | 1.58                |
| 1991     | 9.07                | 2.14                |
| 2001(est.) | 9.39              | 2.57                |

By 2025, over 20 per cent of the population will be aged 65 and over.

As the number of older people living in the community increases, so there will be a corresponding increase in the demand for care ser-vices, in particular home care. Home care is not a cheap option. The

5 CIPFA figures.
6 Government Statistical Service DoH Statistical Bulletin 1998/13.
7 Social Trends (1995).

more complex the range of needs, the more the service will cost to provide.

However, the money available to local authorities to meet the cost of home care is limited, whilst the level of demand for services appears unlimited. This has led local authorities to find ways of controlling the amount of money spent on providing home care, including:

■ Increasing the level and complexity of the requirements for care (known as the eligibility criteria) for which services are provided. People who do not meet the eligibility requirements will either not receive a service or may receive a contribution in the form of a voucher towards purchasing the cost of their care themselves.

■ Prioritising needs and meeting some needs and not others. Some groups of people may be classed as a priority for receiving home care services even if they do not meet the requirements of the eligibility criteria. These are likely to be either family and personal carers who need the support of a paid Home Carer to enable them to continue to provide the major part of the care; or people who are in need of short-term care, for example on discharge from hospital, to enable them to become fully independent again.

■ Placing a cash limit on home care services generally equivalent to the weekly cost of a place in a residential home. This is a form of rationing, placing a ceiling on the cost of the home care that can be provided.

■ Introducing and/or increasing the charge levied for the provision of the service. Only five or six authorities in the country now provide a free service. Most authorities do provide a free service for people on income support, but expect a contribution from people who receive the attendance allowance.

All of these restrictions are designed to obtain 'best value' for money – to target the provision of services to those people who are in greatest need and make the limited amount of money 'stretch' as far as possible. Figures from the Department of Health support this, showing that although overall there has been a significant increase in the number of home care contact hours (up 6 per cent in 1997 on the previous year's figure), there has also been a corresponding decrease in the total number of households receiving home care (down over 4 per cent in 1997)[8] indicating that more home care hours are being provided for fewer people.

As a result there is an increasing emphasis on the provision of personal care services rather than practical care. If you only require assistance with tasks such as cleaning the home or shopping, you are unlikely, in most places in the country, to obtain a service through the social services department, although you may be referred to an organisation such as Age Concern, who can provide a service at a reasonable cost which the customer will have to pay. A few authorities operate a 'voucher' scheme which contributes towards the cost of purchasing practical home care, privately.

To counter-balance this trend, the Government is to introduce a new grant in April 1999 for three years. The 'Promoting Independence: Prevention' grant is designed to target some 'low level' support to people who are assessed as being most at risk of losing their independence.

In addition, as with charging policies, the Government is concerned to ensure greater consistency in the way in which the eligibility criteria are applied, both within the same authority and between different authorities.

## *Provision of 24-hour care*

A further concept associated with the introduction of community care is that of customer choice and developing 'consumer-orientated' services. Given the choice (generally within certain limits defined by the cost), most people want to stay in their own homes as long as possible, rather than enter residential care. This means that the care needs of people living in their own homes is increasing, becoming more complex, more demanding and challenging.

---

8 Government Statistical Service DoH Statistical Bulletin 1998/13.

In order to meet these challenges, home care is now provided by many organisations, including local authority own services, on a 24-hour basis, 365 days a year.

The peak time of care provision has changed from between 9 in the morning and midday to between 7 and 9 in both the mornings and the evenings, reflecting the need for assistance with getting up, washed and dressed and then going to bed.

Ironically the quiet time, as ever, is between 2 pm and 5 pm. No one wants to have personal or practical care in the afternoons, which is one reason why the majority of Home Carers continue to be employed on a part-time basis rather than full-time.

In order to provide cover 24 hours a day, many organisations, including local authority in-house services, have introduced shift working for home care, including split shifts to allow for the quiet period in the afternoon. Shifts may be rotating, or some organisations allow Home Carers to work the same shift on a regular basis to fit in with other home and family circumstances.

The increase in the level of dependency of people needing care and new regulations on manual handling introduced by the European Union[9] mean that it is becoming increasingly common for Home Carers to work in pairs to enable them to lift people and help them in and out of bed and chairs.

The introduction of other schemes such as night checking services, usually linked to community alarm systems, has also proved effective in providing 24-hour care. Government measures to reduce 'bed blocking' in hospitals and to cope with the demand for hospital beds in winter has led to the development of a number of special home care schemes to provide short-term emergency care in the home to people who would otherwise have been admitted to hospital. The development of these innovatory schemes, including more 'joint' provision between health and social care services, will continue into the new millennium.

---

9 Manual Handling Regulations 1992 – European Directive.

As the complexity of the need for care increases, so it is likely that people will receive care from teams of Home Carers, possibly employed by different organisations. For example, one team providing services during the week and another team at weekends. This is not always popular with people needing care, who, as we saw in Chapter 1, prefer to have one or two carers that they can get to know personally.

**In summary** The home care service is changing as demand increases and services have to be rationed. It now generally provides a 24-hour service, 7 days a week, targeted on those people who have the greatest and most complex care needs.

# Modernising social services: promoting independence, improving protection, raising standards

The publication of the White Paper at the end of November 1998 heralded major changes in the way in which social care is provided and sets the scene for taking the provision of social care services into the new millennium. It builds on the changes that have taken place throughout the 1980s and 1990s; seeks to refocus direction where it may have gone off course, for example in meeting the specific needs of individuals; rebalances the emphasis, for example in relation to the need to provide some preventative care to people with low level needs; and plugs gaps, for example the need for regulation of home care.

## *Seven key principles*

The White Paper identifies seven key principles which are at the heart of the modernisation programme. In summary, these are:

1 Care should be provided to people in a way that supports their independence and respects their dignity.
2 Services should meet individuals' specific needs, pulling together the services from across health, social services, housing, etc. People should have a say in what services they get and how they are delivered.

3 Care services should be organised, accessed, provided and financed in a fair, open and consistent way in every part of the country.

4 Children who, for whatever reason, need to be looked after by local authorities should get a decent start in life with the same opportunities to make a success of their life as any other child.

5 Every person, child or adult, should be safeguarded against abuse, neglect or poor treatment whilst receiving care.

6 People who receive social services should have an assurance that the staff they deal with are sufficiently trained and skilled for the work they are doing.

7 People should be able to have confidence in their local social services, knowing that they work to clear and acceptable standards and that if those standards are not met, action can be taken to improve things.

 **What do you think these principles mean for the way in which you work – do you think that they will mean an improvement in the service received by people who need care? How do you think you can contribute to their implementation in practice?**

## Regulation of home care

We touched briefly, earlier in this chapter, on the issue of regulation for home care. The Residential Homes Act 1983 introduced regulation and inspection of all private and voluntary residential and nursing homes. The powers were subsequently extended to include homes run by the local authority social services department. Every home must meet certain criteria to be registered and placed on the approved list of homes and be inspected at least twice a year – once announced and once unannounced.

The principal purpose of the registration and inspection is to protect the physical and mental wellbeing of the people living in the home and ensure their quality of life and standard of living meets acceptable standards.

At the time of writing, there is no equivalent regulation for domiciliary care, even though many of the people receiving care in their own homes, live on their own, are relatively isolated and potentially vulnerable to exploitation. As the law currently stands, anyone may set up a home care service and offer their services to vulnerable people irrespective of whether they have the skills, knowledge and experience of the work, or whether they have a criminal record.

However, the Government is committed to introducing legislation to regulate organisations providing personal care services to people living in their own homes, including local authority in-house services. It is not proposed that regulation will be compulsory, but it is assumed that the majority of organisations will wish to register. The local authority will be able to contract only with registered and regulated agencies for the provision of home care. Those who are registered will be required to display a 'kite mark' to indicate to prospective purchasers of their service, including private purchasers, that they are registered and inspected.

 **What is your view on this? Do you think there should be regulation of organisations providing home care? Virtually everyone involved in home care thinks there should be regulation, and a Bill is likely to be presented to Parliament so that it becomes law early in the new millennium.**

In the meantime, in the absence of national regulation, many local authorities have introduced voluntary regulation schemes and 'approved provider' lists. However, the quality and rigour of the schemes varies greatly.

## Standards for regulation of the organisation

Regulation of home care agencies will be undertaken by the new Commissions for Care Standards (CCSs) – independent, statutory bodies operating in eight regions in England with wide responsibilities for the regulation of care provided for people in residential and nursing homes and in their own homes.

The standards for registration have yet to be developed but are likely to include areas such as:

- The suitability of the owner or manager in relation to the business they are providing.
- Personnel issues, such as recruitment, selection and vetting procedures, criminal record check, policies on health and safety, training and equal opportunities, etc.
- Information provided to the people receiving the service, including charges, withdrawal of service, emergency provision, complaints procedures, etc.
- Quality procedures, including obtaining the views of the people receiving care on the standard of the service, supervision of staff, etc.
- Operational policies, including the administration of medicines, confidentiality, health and safety, access to people's homes, etc.
- Financial viability and insurance.

There will be wide consultation on the development of the standards to ensure that they are generally acceptable and applicable. They will be legally enforceable on the registered organisations.

Police checks on care staff are a difficult area. Almost all application forms ask whether the applicant has a criminal record, but it is generally not possible to check whether the information provided is accurate. Only for work with children is there a statutory requirement to undertake a police check of criminal records – and even then this often takes a long time to complete. In spite of the publicity given to abuse of older people there is currently no compulsory requirement to undertake a police check. This situation is likely to be changed with the introduction of regulation for home care.

## *Standards for regulation of the individual care worker*

There are also proposals to keep a register of individuals accredited to provide care, through what is called the General Social Care Council (GSCC), as we saw in the previous chapter. These proposals have been discussed for the past ten years but should become a reality by the new millennium. Those individuals on the register will be required to follow a code of conduct and practice. Initially the register will only apply to social workers and residential staff working with children, and the current debate is whether and when the register should be extended to include everyone who works in care.

 **What is your view? Do you think you and your colleagues, including your managers, should be on a register as approved providers of care? Again, most people in home care think you should, but what would be the criteria for being on the register? In addition to satisfactory references and police checks, there are likely to be a number of other factors, including a requirement to be trained to a certain level within a specific timespan. In relation to home care, this would be S/NVQ Level 2 as identified in Appendix 1.**

**In summary** The Government is intent on modernising social services and ensuring that it is better equipped to meet the specific needs of individuals and provide them with quality services. Although there is no statutory regulation of either agencies or people providing home care in 1999, this should be in place early in the new millennium.

## The commissioning and contracting process in home care

The information that follows on the commissioning and contracting process only applies when someone is receiving care through their local social services department. This process does not apply to people who have sufficient financial resources to be able to purchase the care they require themselves and who do not need the assistance of social services.

Take another look at the six key objectives for community care on page 32.

Achieving the last four of these objectives, ie 'good care management', 'the development of a flourishing independent sector', 'clarifying the responsibilities of agencies', and 'better value for taxpayers' money' has led in most social services departments to the separation of the process of assessment of the need for care and contracting the service provision from the actual provision of the care itself.

## _Assessment of the need for care_

If you are providing home care services on behalf of the local authority social services department, before you are asked to go into the home of a new customer, a comprehensive assessment of their care needs should have been undertaken, including an assessment of the risks involved in providing the care.

If the care needs are unclear and/or complex, the assessment will generally have been undertaken by a member of staff of the social services department, who may be called a care manager, but may also be given many other job titles. Occasionally the care assessment may be undertaken by a health service professional, particularly if it relates to a discharge from hospital or a complex package of care involving the provision of both health and social care.

If the care needs are straightforward and it is clear that there is a need for home care, the assessment may have been undertaken by a manager in the social services in-house home care service.

The assessment of care needs should be all-embracing and cover all aspects of the care required to support someone in their own home. There should also be an assessment of their financial circumstances including the benefits they receive such as an attendance allowance and whether they are on income support. The financial assessment will indicate whether the person is able to contribute towards the cost of providing their care. Most importantly at this stage, it should also include an assessment of the risks involved in delivering the care in the home, as this will affect the work that you do and the nature of the 'care package' that is provided to the person concerned. (More information about risk is given in Chapter 7, 'Health and Safety'.)

The NHS and Community Care Act 1990 was designed to ensure that people with care needs and their relatives are involved in decisions relating to the care they receive and that, wherever possible and practicable, they are given choice in the nature of and way in which the care services are provided. This is part of what is known as developing a 'needs-led' approach rather than 'service-led'. This means that the person receiving care is the focus and that the care services you provide should be those specifically required by that person and in line with the local authority's priorities (needs-led), not those which either the organisation you work for or the social services department that has assessed the needs decides are available (service-led). This principle is repeated in the 1998 White Paper, *Modernising Social Services*:

> 'Everyone deserves to be treated as an individual and to have the system geared to their needs, not vice versa.'

The outcome of the care assessment is written up in a care plan. This should have been discussed with the person concerned and any family carer and their agreement obtained to the ways in which the care plan will be met.

You may find that some people you care for do not have a care plan. These should generally be people who entered the system before the implementation of the NHS and Community Care Act. If you think someone you are caring for should have a care plan, or you think that they need a reassessment of their care, refer it to your line manager, who in turn should refer the person to a care manager or similar person responsible for the assessment of care needs.

*Modernising Social Services* emphasises the need for regular reviews and follow-ups to the original assessment. This is something that, under pressure of work, has often fallen by the wayside in the past until an emergency situation has triggered a reassessment. In future, reviews should be undertaken after three months and annually thereafter unless circumstances require an earlier review. Since providers may play a part in the reviews, you may find you are involved in assisting in a review of someone for whom you are providing care.

## Components of the care plan

Some or all of the following information should be included in the care plan that is compiled for each person. The exact content of the plan will vary depending upon the assessed care needs of individuals and the complexity of the plan, but will normally include the following:

- Assessed care needs, including the abilities and capabilities of each person.
- Priorities in meeting care needs. **Note** There may well be care needs which are of low priority and are therefore not met.
- How the care needs will be met.
- Others involved, including family carers and health staff, and when.
- Principal points of contact (family, care manager and service-providing organisation).
- Any particular medical conditions of which it is necessary for service providers to be aware.
- Any special dietary requirements.
- Individual personal preferences that affect the provision of care.
- Outcome from the risk assessment, including any health and safety hazards that have been identified.
- Ways of maintaining and supporting independence and acknowledged risks that have been identified.
- Individual outcomes required from the care package.

A copy of the care plan should be left with the person who is receiving the service. You also should have access to the care plan and be able to see it to ensure you are providing all the care that is required and are working towards the outcomes identified but are not going beyond your duties. You also need to know what other organisations (if any) are also providing care services to the same person, so that you can coordinate the visits to the home and the provision of care.

## Commissioning the provision of care

Once the care needs have been identified and the care plan agreed with the person needing care, the next stage is to commission the provision of care. This may be a simple, straightforward process in which the person responsible for commissioning the care approaches a number of service providers to see whether they are able to provide the care required at the right price; or it may be a more complicated process.

Unless you only provide care to people who are able to meet the full cost themselves, the care you provide will almost certainly be part of a contract between the local authority social services department as the 'commissioner' and purchaser of services on behalf of the person needing care, and your employing organisation (including local authority 'in-house' home care services) as the provider of services. This separation of functions is often referred to as the 'purchaser/provider split'.

Your line manager will want to be sure that you provide care to the standard required and within the costs specified in the contract and that the work you undertake does not break or go beyond conditions of the 'contract' in any way. There will, however, be some flexibility in the contract in case of emergencies, for example if the person you are caring for has had an accident and you have to stay with them until an ambulance arrives.

Local authority social services departments are seeking 'best value' for the money they spend and will be monitoring the contract that they place with your employing organisation to ensure that all the conditions are met. This will include, for example, ensuring that if they purchase one hour of care, that is what the person receives, and not 40 minutes. Various forms of 'swipe' cards and other mechanisms for checking the time spent and the activities undertaken will be introduced by most authorities over the next few years.

**In summary** The commissioning and contracting process is illustrated in the diagrams opposite.

## Complaints procedure

The National Health Service and Community Care Act 1990 required all social services departments to put in place and publicise a formal complaints procedure, to try to ensure that complaints from people needing care and their families are investigated and dealt with in a structured and positive way. The intention is that a proper complaints procedure can provide safeguards and protection both for people receiving care services and, in the case of unjustified or malicious complaints, for staff.

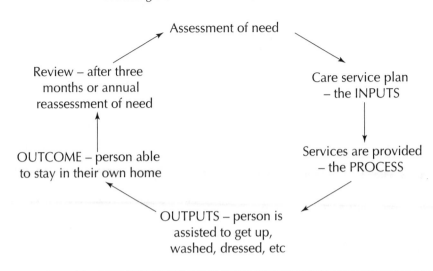

Assessment of need

Review – after three months or annual reassessment of need

Care service plan – the INPUTS

OUTCOME – person able to stay in their own home

Services are provided – the PROCESS

OUTPUTS – person is assisted to get up, washed, dressed, etc

Person is referred to social services for care at home

Allocated to a care manager or the equivalent

Care assessment undertaken including a risk assessment and a financial assessment

Care plan compiled, discussed and agreed with person needing care

Care providers approached to deliver care package

Contract placed with provider organisation

You start work to provide the care required

Although only social services departments have to have formal complaints procedures by law, it has become increasingly necessary for voluntary organisations and private agencies to have their own complaints procedures. This may be written into the contract with social services and is now considered to be an indication of good practice.

You need to obtain a copy of your employing organisation's complaints procedure. If they do not have one, you might like to show them this book and suggest they should! If you work for a private or voluntary organisation, you may find it useful to have a copy of your local social services department's complaints procedure, since this may also be used by the people you are caring for and their families.

All your customers should have been informed of the procedure for making a complaint, both when agreeing the care plan and when visited for the first time by your line manager.

If you follow the guidance in this book, it is unlikely, but not impossible, that any of the people you are caring for will make a complaint against you and the service you are providing. Nevertheless, you do need to be well informed about the complaints procedure.

Remember that a person who has difficulty seeing properly and has sight problems may not be fully aware of the complaints procedure. They should be encouraged to seek information from the social services department or from your employer and ask for it to be sent to them in a suitable form such as an audio tape or Braille.

In reality, the vast majority of complaints about the provision of care to people in their own homes relate to differences of opinion on the assessment of need between the professionals on one hand and the person needing care and/or their family on the other. Although every effort will be made to resolve such differences of opinion, at the end of the day the complaints procedure is the last course of action. As a Home Carer, you must be aware of this, if any of the people you are caring for find themselves in this situation.

Don't resist complaints. They can help you provide a better service. However, as the Home Carer you will often be the first person, on the spot, able to put things right before they become a formal complaint. Putting things right first time can often save a lot of work, worry and anxiety later. A complaint should become formal only after all informal channels to solve the problem have been exhausted.

 **Think how you will feel if someone you are caring for complains about what you are doing or how you are doing it. What action will you take?**

It is important to recognise that a small number of people always complain about everything. There will be nothing you can do to please or satisfy them. In these circumstances, the formal complaints procedure is there to protect you as well.

Always inform your line manager if you think a complaint may be made against you, for whatever reason. If you are a member of a trade union, they may also be able to help you. If you have provided the care services to the standard specified, you should have nothing to fear.

## Components of a complaints procedure

Typical components of a complaints policy are that it should:

- be well defined and publicised;
- define exactly what a complaint is;
- recognise that users have a right to challenge decisions made by the agency and information held about them;
- be part of, and not a substitute for, good practice.

## The procedure itself

The complaints procedure should:

- recognise that service users may be vulnerable and/or powerless and, as a result, afraid to use a complaints procedure;
- allow for and encourage service users to make use of advocates (ie independent people who will help them make out their case or

speak on their behalf and represent their interests);
- be part of the organisation and not 'added on' to it;
- be simple to understand and to operate;
- involve staff, and unions (if appropriate), and allow them to give their views;
- indicate where and when criminal proceedings are appropriate;
- recognise that some users will not complain, despite having a good cause or reason (lack of complaints may not be an indication that all is well but, rather, that people find it difficult to complain – this particularly applies to home care).

 **Obtain a copy of your organisation's complaints procedure and consider the extent to which it meets these criteria.**

**In summary** It is good practice for all organisations to have a formal complaints procedure. It is there to protect people needing care and the staff providing the care. Your customers should be aware of the procedure or know from where they can obtain information on it.

# The interface with health services

In the late 1990s and into the new century, the lines of responsibility between health and social care services in the provision of home care will become increasingly blurred, possibly leading eventually to some form of amalgamation – although this has been ruled out for the time being.

There are a number of reasons why health and social care will move closer together, some of which are given below:

- Many of the people you are caring for have complex needs and will be visited regularly by health staff such as community or district nurses as well as by Home Carers. With you, they will form a multi-disciplinary care team.
- Continuing care for people who have been in hospital and are terminally – but not acutely – ill, will take place in their own homes as well as in nursing and residential homes.
- Advances in surgical techniques mean that people can attend a

day hospital or be discharged early from hospital to recover at home. This has already led to an expansion in 'hospital at home' schemes.

■ Closure of long-stay hospitals for people with learning disabilities and people with mental health problems and their resettlement in ordinary homes in the community, with appropriate support from care teams including home care.

■ The development of special schemes such as those mentioned earlier to alleviate 'winter pressures' and reduce the demand for beds in acute hospitals.

The boundaries between community and primary health care and social care are becoming increasingly blurred. Community health care has much more in common with social care than with most acute (hospital) care. Successive Government policies in 1998 relating specifically to health, but including social care, such as the Health Improvement Programmes (HImPs) and Health Action Zones (HAZs) contribute further to breaking down the boundaries between health and social care which have existed since the introduction of the NHS in 1948.

The care of people with learning disabilities or mental health problems, living in the community, is already leading to the establishment of specialist home care teams, trained to meet the particular needs of these people. The nature of the care they require is different in that a major component will be training the service user to undertake tasks for themselves and enabling them to maximise their own potential.

Other specialist schemes caring for people in their own homes include:

■ Night-sitting service when a person needs someone in attendance at night.

■ Discharge from hospital – a more intensive service for people who have been discharged early or need to ease the move from hospital to home.

■ Out-of-hours service for people who need care early morning, at night or at weekends.

- Respite service – ranging from a few hours to 24-hour care to give the personal family carer a break.
- Emergency service to prevent unnecessary admission to hospital when a crisis occurs.

These schemes may be run jointly by the local community health trust and social services or by one or other agency. If you are not directly involved in these specialist schemes yourself, find out which schemes operate in your area, so that you can give advice if necessary.

The present Government places considerable emphasis on working in partnership, across boundaries, particularly in relation to the health service. Additional 'winter pressures' money for joint health and social care initiatives has been made available in 1997/98 and in 1998/99 to help ease pressure on the health and social care system. The Government also proposes legislation to make it easier for health and social services to work together. Three key proposals include:

1 Pooled budgets – to facilitate the provision of more integrated care.
2 Lead commissioning- where the transfer of funds from one body to the other enables the organisation receiving the funds to purchase services on behalf of both bodies.
3 Integrated provision – where one organisation provides both the health and the social care services.

This last proposal could potentially have a significant impact on the provision of home care, rationalising the number of people who may enter the home to provide the care.

As we move towards the new century, the role and function of health staff working in the community, including nurses and care staff and social services staff, must come closer together and in some instances, combine. After all, it makes little sense to have one set of staff come into a home to assist the person with getting up, washed and dressed, and someone else to come along to change a dressing or give an injection. In time it may become the norm to access home care through your local GP practice. The introduction of Primary Care Groups (PCGs) – groupings of doctors generally serving a local population of 100,000 people or more – in 1999 is very likely to lead in time to the provision of a wide range of other health and social care services through the PCG, including home care.

**In summary** The current division between community and primary health care and social care will gradually be eroded and in the long term is probably not sustainable. In the meantime, there will need to be close cooperation between Home Carers and health staff

# Introduction of Direct Payments

The Community Care (Direct Payments) Act was passed in 1996 and came into effect in 1997. This enables social services to assess the care needs of adults aged under 65 and then provide the person needing care with the financial resources to purchase their own care.

At present the Act does not apply to people aged 65 and over. However, the Government have undertaken to withdraw the age limitation so that people aged 65 and over are eligible to receive Direct Payments. It is therefore possible that by the start of the new millennium, many people (or their family or independent advocate on their behalf) may be responsible for purchasing their own care from a wide range of providing organisations.

The Act enables people who are unable to meet the full cost of their care themselves, be responsible for and manage their own care in the same way as people who can meet the cost themselves and do not need assistance from social services. The Act raises a number of issues including, for example, how people in receipt of Direct Payments will decide on who to purchase the care from, particularly when there is no system in place for registering or accrediting all organisations or individuals providing care. At the time of writing, the inter-relationship between the intention of the Government to extend Direct Payments to people aged over 65 and the proposals for the registration and regulation of organisations providing home care, which falls short of requiring all organisations providing personal care to be registered, is unclear. Hopefully this will shortly be clarified.

> **Q** What do you think about the Act? Do you think Direct Payments are a good idea and do you think they should be extended to people aged 65 and over? Do you think it will change the nature of your relationship with your customers in any way?

**In summary** The Community Care (Direct Payments) Act currently only applies to adults aged under 65 but will be extended to include people aged 65+ in the future.

# Development and training of Home Carers

In the past, the majority of Home Carers have received relatively little in the way of training and personal development, in spite of the importance of the work in caring for vulnerable people. This situation cannot be allowed to continue into the next century. As the work of a Home Carer becomes more complex, you are unlikely to be fully effective as a Home Carer or be able to perform the tasks identified in this book, competently, unless you have received the appropriate training.

Appendix 1 identifies the units related to the Level 2 Scottish National Vocational Qualification (S/NVQ) award in Care. That is the ideal training for the work that you will undertake. However, it may not be immediately available to you, although this book should help you prepare and work towards it. Each chapter identifies the units to which it relates.

Funding for S/NVQ Level 2 and key skills is available from some TECS (Training and Education Councils) for National Traineeships in health and social care, provided trainees complete the training by their 25th birthday. This may also be available for existing employees.

If you are unable to work towards your S/NVQ in the short term, you should be provided with essential in-house training by your employing organisation. All employers should provide you with induction training on the key topics, followed by further training on other essential areas as well as expanding the topics covered in induction. Training which should be available to you should include the following:

## *Induction*

- Basic values that should underpin the provision of care.
- The provision of non-discriminatory services and practice.
- Health and safety.
- Moving and handling.
- Standards to be attained in the delivery of services.
- Communication skills – including people who are hearing impaired.
- Basic first aid, including hypothermia.

### Essential:

- The process of ageing.
- Common disabilities and diseases.
- Awareness of the effect of visual impairment (partial sight).

### Desirable:

- Maintaining continence.
- Dealing with aggressive behaviour.
- Caring for confused people.

## *Specialist training*

- Caring for people who are terminally ill.
- Caring for people from ethnic minority communities – their particular needs.
- The tasks of a nursing auxiliary (eg changing dressings; pressure sores).
- Caring for people with learning disabilities.
- Caring for people with mental health problems.
- Working in dirty and/or infested homes.

At the end of the day, community care, providing care for vulnerable people in their own homes, can succeed only if you, the Home Carer, have the skills, abilities and commitment to undertake your part of the care plan for each person that you are caring for and ensure that they receive a high-quality service. That requires effective training.

Undertaking necessary training is likely to be one of the standards for regulating home care organisations and a requirement for individual registration with the General Social Care Council.

## *The need for personal support*

The Home Carer is the person who is most frequently in contact with the person requiring care and knows more about them and their care needs than anyone else within the care agencies. Organisations providing care overlook the views and needs of the Home Carer at their peril.

Most Home Carers work on their own in other people's homes. However, as we have said earlier, they should not be working in isolation. The Home Carer should be provided with, or have access to the following support, through their employing agency:

- Support, for example from other Home Carers and from workers from other agencies carrying out similar or complementary tasks.
- Regular, structured supervision from immediate supervisor/manager/organiser (unless registered self-employed).
- Contract of employment and a job description (unless registered self-employed).
- Clear policies, procedures and a code of practice to which they are expected to work.
- A system of obtaining help in an emergency.
- A system of obtaining help and advice at any other time.
- Colleagues and managers at work who will listen to Home Carers and take their views and opinions into account and recognise the stress that occurs in the work.
- Managers who value Home Carers and their work, monitor their progress and give them feedback on their performance.

*Q*  **Is there anything else you would add to this list?**

Appendix 3 gives further information that should be provided for Home Carers, on the organisation's policies and practices.

If you are provided with the appropriate and necessary training opportunities and support from your line manager and colleagues, you will be in a position to provide the service your customers need to the standard required, into the next century.

**In summary** It is essential that you receive induction training before commencing work. You should also have the opportunity to work towards obtaining your S/NVQ Level 2 award in Care. You should also be provided with support and supervision on an on-going basis.

## CASE STUDY

### Mark, aged 30 years

In 1984, Mark was an easy-going, friendly and popular young man of 17 years of age. He had left school and was a trainee chef at a hotel not far from his home. One morning he left work in the early hours on his motorcycle which slipped on the wet leaves in the drive.

He was discovered lying on the ground. He had fallen and hit his head, bursting a blood vessel in his brain. The accident left him in a coma for two months and wheelchair-bound for 13 years until he died in 1997.

Eighteen months after his accident, Mark came home to live with his parents. The hard work of caring for Mark had begun, 24 hours a day, 7 days a week. Mark could hardly move his arms or legs, eat, drink or talk, in fact anything that required the use of his muscles.

Mark and his parents were referred for home care service on his return home. Initially 11 years ago, the service primarily focused on domestic tasks. As the service changed so did the type of service provided to Mark and his parents.

Mark's mother continued to care for Mark but was wearing herself out in the process. Home Carers began to work alongside her assisting with Mark's personal care.

Mark's mother's health deteriorated and it was agreed two Home Carers would attend Mark every morning. They arrived at 8.30 am and spent 1½ hours with Mark, washing, bathing, dressing and feeding him. Home Carers attended again in the evening to assist Mark in getting ready for bed.

Mark's mother developed confidence and trust in the staff who attended and she would often take the opportunity to take the family dog for a walk whilst the Home Carers cared for her son.

## QUESTIONS

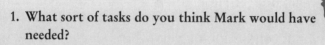

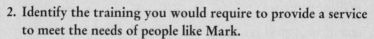

1. What sort of tasks do you think Mark would have needed?

2. Identify the training you would require to provide a service to meet the needs of people like Mark.

3. What do you think would be the needs of Mark's mother and how would you respond to these needs?

4. What do you think would be the major difference between working on your own and working with someone else?

## KEY POINTS

- Milestones in the development of the home care service include the 1948 National Health and National Assistance Act and the 1990 NHS and Community Care Act.
- One of the major outcomes of the NHS and Community Care Act has been a shift in emphasis towards home care rather than residential care.
- There has been major growth in the number of private and voluntary sector organisations providing home care.
- The demand and need for home care services is greater than the resources available to meet the needs. This has led to tightening up of the eligibility criteria and rationing. Only those with the most complex care needs generally now receive help.

- The home care market in England alone was worth £1,028.1 million in 1995.
- Care is now provided in most parts of the country 24 hours a day, 7 days a week.
- *Modernising Social Services* is the Government White Paper which was published at the end of 1998 and sets the agenda for social services into the new millennium.
- Included in the White Paper are proposals to introduce long-awaited legislation to regulate home care agencies.
- The establishment of the General Social Care Council will introduce codes of conduct and practice and register individual care workers, starting with those working with children and families.
- Home Carers should be aware of the contents of the care plan, including the risk assessment, drawn up for each person as a result of assessment of their care needs.
- Wherever possible, people needing care and their families should be involved in decisions about the home care they receive and, when possible, given choices in the sort of care and the way in which it is provided.
- Home Carers should also be aware in general terms of any conditions within the contract to provide services, between their employing organisation/unit and the social services department purchasing the service, that will affect the way in which they do their work.
- Make sure you obtain a copy of your organisation's complaints procedure and that of your local social services department if it is different. Some, if not all, of the people you are caring for will be aware of it and may use it.
- Over time the boundaries between health care and social care will gradually be eroded. It may become more common to access social care as well as health care through GP practices and health centres.
- The current age limit of 65 on Direct Payments to adults is to be removed.
- In order to deliver the quality services people should expect, you must be provided with appropriate training and personal support by your employing organisation.

# 4  The Health of Older People

S/NVQ Level 2: This chapter relates to the mandatory units O1, CL1 and Z1; Option Group A units W2, W3, Z7, Z9, Z19; Option Group B units CU3, W8, Y1, Z8.

Many of the people you will care for in their own homes will be in need of care because they are mentally and/or physically frail. This applies particularly to very old people, who tend to become more susceptible to illness the longer they live. This chapter introduces you to the ageing process and to some of the more common illnesses of later life. It discusses ways of maintaining the health of the older person, including the need for social and emotional care and sexual expression. The chapter also explores particular issues in relation to medication and caring for people who have challenging behaviour or refuse to care for themselves.

## Changes in the body and common problems

Simply being old does not in itself make a person ill or disabled. Even when ageing is partly responsible for a problem, treatment is very often still possible. Remember that the Queen Mother had two hip replacements in her late 90s! You should do everything you can to encourage the older people you care for to seek help for medical and health problems, and not just to put it down to 'old age'.

The changes described below are due partly to ageing and partly to disease. As the body ages:

- The skin becomes drier and more wrinkled, and brown spots may appear on the backs of the hands. Finger and toenails thicken and become more brittle. Hair becomes grey and thins; early greying and baldness run in families. People may 'shrink', becoming shorter, because the discs between the vertebrae become thinner and also because of bone changes.

- Bones become thinner and more brittle (osteoporosis) and may also lose calcium; they therefore break more easily. Softened vertebrae may be crushed by the weight they carry. This painful process bends the spine, so the person becomes stooped. Bone changes happen much faster in women than in men, but can be slowed down by hormone replacement therapy.

- Muscles become less powerful and joints less supple. These changes can be much less in people who keep active and take exercise. Inactive old people become progressively less and less mobile.

- Balance and coordination deteriorate. This can make older people more likely to fall over, especially if they have health problems or the home is unsafe.

- Older people are at risk from extremes of temperature because their body's temperature-control mechanisms become less efficient.

- Hearing may be impaired, especially with group conversations, in noisy surroundings or when speech is distorted (eg by a public address system in railway station announcements). Hearing-impaired people may be thought to be confused if their hearing problem is not identified. Treatment or a hearing aid may help.

- As the lens of the eye loses focusing power, spectacles become necessary for close work such as reading; this is quite normal. However, two out of five people over 75 years old have sight problems affecting their independence and enjoyment of life. This is abnormal and should be investigated. Common causes are cataracts, macular degeneration, glaucoma and diabetes. Treatment can prevent or halt sight loss; in addition, the affected person can be helped to make the most of their remaining sight.

- Taste and smell become less acute. This may reduce the older person's enjoyment of food.

- Teeth may be lost because of gum disease, and dentures work loose as gums shrink. Good dental care with frequent check-ups can keep teeth healthy for life. People with dentures should have them checked once a year.

- Incontinence of urine and/or stool can develop. This is not due to ageing alone, and it can often be successfully treated.
- Older people often suffer from constipation. Fibre in the diet, plenty of fluids and adequate exercise can prevent this.
- The lungs and airways become less efficient. Heart and blood vessel disease becomes more common and blood pressure tends to rise. Older people are more likely to suffer from strokes, chest infections, arthritis, diabetes and cancer than younger people are.

**Remember** that no one older person will suffer from all or even most of these conditions.

**Never** assume that getting older automatically makes someone disabled or ill.

**Always** treat people according to their condition and not according to their age.

 **Think about some of the older people you know. How many would you consider to be fit and active? How many would you describe as being 'young in spirit'? Now think about some younger people. Would you describe any of these as being 'old before their time'? Why do you think this has happened?**

We can therefore make some important points about the ageing process that you should always keep in mind when you are providing care:

- People can age at different rates. Some people in their 70s can appear to be in their 50s, and vice versa.
- Never assume that an older person can't improve both mentally and physically.
- A healthy lifestyle can prevent or delay some of the illnesses that can affect older people. The most important thing is not to smoke; it is never too late for a person's health to benefit from giving up.
- Regular exercise helps to keep older people active. Eating a good variety of foods, with plenty of fibre, fruit and vegetables, and

fluids also helps. The possible link between animal fats and heart disease is less important in later life.

- Never equate old age with ill health or disabilities. If you treat older people as if they are ill, they may respond by letting you do everything for them, and so losing the ability to do whatever they can for themselves. The majority of people aged over 70 are very fit and active. However, they are unlikely to be receiving home care services. The people you care for will be frailer than average and not typical of older people as a group.
- Do not patronise or 'talk down' to adults about their health or disabilities. Phrases such as 'How are we today then?' should be avoided, however kindly they are meant.
- Maintain strict confidentiality about what you know about a person's medical condition, or, for that matter, about anything else you might know about him or her. The only exception to the rule is when you may need to report to a GP, district nurse or other health professional, including your line manager, on any matters that concern the person receiving care.

Keep in mind that people should **never** be described as if they were illnesses. People are not 'diabetics', 'epileptics' or 'schizophrenics.' They are people first and foremost who happen to have diabetes, epilepsy or schizophrenia. The emphasis must always be on the person, not on the illness.

Appendix 7 lists the more common illnesses and disabilities that may affect older people. Some of these conditions are preventable, whilst others can improve or be kept stable with proper care. Some are progressive, and then treatment aims to keep the sufferer as comfortable as possible. The aim of care is to keep people in good health and to make sure that any disabilities interfere with their lives as little as possible.

**In summary** The vast majority of people aged over 70 are fit and active. You should do whatever you can to encourage the people you care for to seek medical help to improve their physical and/or mental health and not just put problems down to 'old age'.

# Social and emotional care

In order to maintain the health of the older person you must take into account their social and emotional needs as well as their physical needs. Personal care becomes superficial if the sole concern is for physical needs. This is known as caring for 'the whole person' and in practice all three – physical, social and emotional care – cannot be separated. The provision of personal care, for example helping someone get up, washed and dressed, can be an excellent opportunity to establish a rapport with the person you are caring for, and develop trust. However, the current trend for very short visits of 15–20 minutes allows little time to establish a rapport and can leave the individual feeling more like an object than a person in their own right.

It is important to get to know the people you are caring for as individuals, their likes and dislikes, their skills, interests and experiences. You can be an important link in helping them to retain contact with people and activities outside of their home.

In Chapter 1 we considered the importance of effective communication in establishing a relationship with the person you are caring for. Good communication is the vital ingredient in meeting people's social and emotional needs.

Conversation with the person receiving care is just as important in maintaining their health and their morale as undertaking the physical tasks. It is important that you spend time talking to the person you are caring for, and building up a relationship.

Research undertaken with people receiving home care in 1996/97[10] found that most people wanted to talk about their personal problems from time to time – generally when something was worrying them. The skill you need to acquire as a Home Carer is to know when the person you are caring for wants to talk about their personal problems, and equally importantly – when they don't.

---

10 'Caring for Competence' JICC Home Care Quality Audit.

They may be suffering from a sense of loss from a recent bereavement and need to talk about it. Be sympathetic and understanding. It is a very bad thing for a bereaved person not to be allowed to talk about the loss of a loved one and to have to 'bottle it up' inside themselves. It would be much better if they were encouraged to share their problem or concern with you, the Home Carer. Helping people talk about their feelings is important.

However, the same research also found that very few people receiving care wanted to hear gossip or about the Home Carer's own personal problems.

Reminiscing about the past is another natural and healthy activity and is often used as a means of reorientating people who show signs of confusion. There is much of interest to be learned from the life experiences of an older person.

However, do not assume that older people have no interest in matters of today. A lively interest in current affairs should be encouraged. The research referred to earlier also showed that the majority of people want to talk to their Home Carer about what is happening in the world and current affairs. People who are housebound particularly may experience the loss of involvement in the outside world, and a general feeling of isolation and being unable to participate. Bringing in a newspaper and discussing what is happening can help reduce their sense of isolation.

People may become housebound not because they are immobile but because of disabilities such as poor sight. Apart from their difficulty in getting about, people with a visual handicap may lack information about local activities because they are unable to read newspapers, etc. You can help overcome these difficulties by telling them about events and finding ways of helping them get out, perhaps with the assistance of volunteers.

Helping to overcome loneliness and loss is vital. People become withdrawn, sleepy, depressed and anxious. Frequently they have problems sleeping and a decreased appetite. Severe depression can often be treated by medication or counselling. The Home Carer is in an ideal position to recognise these symptoms and take appropriate action to alleviate them, including reporting the symptoms to the line manager, GP or district nurse.

It is essential that time and energy are spent trying to improve the value and quality of a person's life. It is worth stressing that, no matter how dependent and frail a person may become, day activities and a social life should be considered as part of their general health and wellbeing. Regularly ask questions such as: 'Is there anything that you would particularly like to do today?' Maybe with help some things can be achieved. Where this is not possible, perhaps the opportunity to talk about 'What I would do if only ...' would ease the frustration.

Action you can take to reduce social and emotional isolation:

- Discover each person's special interests.
- Try to encourage activities that are related to past pleasures.
- Assist in the writing of letters, making telephone calls, arranging visits.
- Discover whether assistance is required to continue lifelong hobbies.
- Encourage relatives, friends, visitors, outings and general contact with the outside world.
- Seek the involvement of the local community and voluntary organisations wherever possible.
- Religious beliefs may have been significant in the person's life. Where possible, help them to continue participating in meetings, services, ceremonies, etc, or ask the appropriate religious leader to visit.
- Aids are available to help with activities; for example, large print books, craft materials and talking books (audio tapes).
- Many areas of the country are served by mobile libraries which enable people to choose their own books. They also generally stock books with large type and talking books (audio tapes) for people with sight problems.

People from ethnic minority communities may be particularly isolated, and effort should be made to put them in contact with the appropriate community groups.

Personal family carers should be put in touch with the local carers' support group, if they have not already contacted them.

 **Can you think of other ways of stimulating a person's interest in life and involving them in activities? What do you think you would do if you found yourself in this position? How would you react? What would you do to fill your time?**

**In summary** It is as important to care for the person's emotional and social health as it is to care for their physical health. The first will in turn affect their general wellbeing and their physical health.

# Changes in health

We have emphasised that you as the Home Carer will frequently be the person who is in the most regular contact with the person you are caring for, and therefore best placed to notice any changes in their physical or mental health which may require medical help or intervention or a reassessment of their care needs.

You therefore need to develop the skill of (unobtrusive) observation, to note any physical or mental changes over time, which might indicate deterioration in health. Typical signs include the following:

- clumsiness of fingers;
- confusion;
- deterioration of hearing or sight;
- dizziness;
- loss of appetite;
- loss of mobility;
- memory loss;
- mood changes;
- shakiness.

Any such symptoms should always be noted and, with the person's (or their carer's) consent, reported to the doctor or district nurse. It may be the policy of your employer that you should inform your line manager – check what the policy and procedure are.

Medical matters should always be discussed in private, but ask people how they feel and encourage them to talk about their symptoms. If necessary or appropriate, discuss with them whether they need to see a doctor. If you have the slightest cause for concern, this should be reported to your line manager.

Encourage annual dental checks, testing of eyesight every two years and hearing checks whenever necessary. Make sure that items such as hearing aids and dentures are regularly cleaned. Arrangements can often be made for dentists, opticians and hearing therapists to visit people in their own home. Your local community health trust should be able to advise you on this.

Diet is important in maintaining health. This is covered in detail in Chapter 8, 'Eating and Nutrition'.

**In summary** Home Carers are often the people who are most likely to notice any change in the physical or mental health of the person they are caring for. You should always report any changes to your line manager and take appropriate action such as contacting the GP or community nurse – with the permission of the person receiving care.

## The effects of cold and low temperatures

The average winter temperature indoors is 18–24° Celsius (64–75° Fahrenheit). If the temperature falls below 16°C (61°F), people have reduced resistance to respiratory infections. Below 12°C (54°F) there is an increase in blood pressure and in the viscosity ('stickiness' and 'thickness') of blood, and below 9°C (48°F) the deep body temperature falls after two or more hours. It has been estimated that for every degree Celsius the winter is colder than average there are 8,000 'excess deaths' in the United Kingdom, the death rate increasing sharply from the age of 65. As a result of low temperatures, older people are particularly at risk from respiratory problems, stroke, heart attack and hypothermia.

The body temperature becomes abnormally low because the body's controlling mechanisms do not work as effectively in old, or very young, people. Hypothermia, if not treated, can lead to unconsciousness and death. Age Concern can often provide thermometers so that an eye can be kept on the temperature.

The Government has introduced special 'Cold Weather' payments to people in receipt of specific benefits to enable them to meet the cost of heating bills. You should be aware of when such payments have been 'triggered' and be able to advise the people you are caring for on how to obtain them.

The Department of Health has a special information and advice telephone line on 'winter warmth'. Many older people live in old homes in which the heating may be relatively inefficient and expensive to run. You should inform your line manager if you think anyone you care for is in this position. They will be able to liaise with other agencies, such as Age Concern, who may be able to help.

Factors which can contribute to the onset of hypothermia include:

- immobility (for whatever reason);
- low income – causing fear of using heating systems to their full effect because of the cost;
- a tendency to fall, particularly if unable to get up from the floor;
- alcohol abuse;
- some mental illnesses and the medicines used to treat them;
- living alone, with no visitors.

Symptoms of hypothermia include:

- coldness and puffy face and skin, cold to the touch;
- coldness of unexposed skin (eg armpit);
- drowsiness;
- mental confusion;
- slurred speech;
- unsteady movement.

You should be aware of the danger of hypothermia and advise the people you are caring for on how to avoid the risk. You can obtain leaflets from your local GP.

If you arrive at a person's home and you suspect that they may be suffering from hypothermia:

1 Immediately contact their GP.
2 Wrap the person in blankets.
3 Turn the heating on or up.
4 If blankets or warm clothing are not available, aluminium foil or newspapers are effective in preventing further heat loss.

Do not move the person from their position.

Do not attempt to apply direct heat to the skin by rubbing or use of a hot water bottle.

**In summary** Watch out for signs of hypothermia and be aware of the appropriate action you should take.

# Assisting with medication

Many of the people you are caring for live on their own and need assistance with taking medication. Home Carers are frequently asked to assist by GPs and community nurses, simply because they are the people who are most frequently in contact with the person needing care. You should never take on this responsibility without first seeking the advice and agreement of your line manager and without undertaking the appropriate training.

Your employing organisation should have a policy on medication and clear guidelines for you, the Home Carer, to follow. The guidelines should include the limitations of the Home Carer's role and responsibility and information on the position with regard to insurance and personal liability. If you are self-employed and do not possess a nursing qualification, you will need to check out the position with your insurance company.

If helping with medicines is part of your job, it will usually be medicines taken by mouth or by inhalation that will concern you. Injected drugs or suppositories should be given only by trained staff such as nurses, or occasionally by properly instructed family members. You should always follow the instructions printed on the bottle or box. Ask advice from the doctor or pharmacist if you do not know what to do. Never alter the treatment plan even at the request of the person you are caring for, without taking advice; for instance, you should never give a double dose of a medicine if one dose has been missed.

If you are asked to apply ointment or cream it is advisable to get the agreement of the person you are caring for or their personal family carer, in writing, and this should be placed on the person's record or file.

All medicines which are taken should be recorded on a medication chart which is kept in the person's home. You should always check the chart to ensure that the medication has not been changed and that the medication has not already been administered.

All medicines should be clearly labelled with the person's name, the name of the drug, the dosage and the 'use by' date. Always check the date; any medication which has expired should be reported to your line manager.

If there is a problem with administering medication, you will probably find the local pharmacist very helpful – but don't contact them without clearing it first with your line manager. Some home care organisations retain the services of a pharmacist to advise them on safe practice in the handling of medication.

A community pharmacy service is evolving in which pharmacists take a more active role in helping people living in their own homes to manage their own medication. Many high users of medication are unable to access a pharmaceutical service themselves and rely on others to do it on their behalf. Pharmacists are now beginning to take direct responsibility themselves, for example for home deliveries of prescriptions, which may alleviate the role that Home Carers have assumed, in the absence of any other responsible person. You will need to find out whether pharmacists in the localities in which you work offer this more pro-active service.

Various forms of monitored dosage systems (MDS) are now available which can be filled once a day or even once a week, and release the medication in the stated dosage at the time of day it is to be taken. The most common form of these is known as a 'Dosset' box.

If your job description forbids you to help with medicines, you should not do so. If you are asked to give this sort of help, you should refuse politely and firmly, and refer the person who has asked you to your line manager for further discussion. In some cases you may find it difficult to follow policy instructions, perhaps because circumstances have changed since decisions were made. If this is so, you should arrange to discuss the situation with your line manager, so that you can explain your difficulties and new guidelines can be laid down if appropriate.

**In summary** Always follow the policy and guidelines of your employing organisation in relation to administering medication. If you are self-employed you need to be aware of the risks involved if you do not have a nursing or equivalent qualification.

# Discharge from hospital

It is in the area of discharge from hospital that the boundaries between health care and social care become extremely blurred, and this will affect the work you do as a Home Carer. It is not only your role that becomes blurred, so does the issue about who pays for the care. Hospital care is free, but a charge is generally made for social care. Many people are now cared for at home – and at a cost, who would have previously been cared for in hospital – for free.

Advances in medicine, less invasive surgical techniques, the closure of long-stay hospital beds, the pressure to shorten the queues of people waiting for operations and an increase in demand for operations are all reasons why people are staying for shorter periods in hospital and are discharged to recover in a nursing home or in their own homes. This trend is likely to continue and possibly increase.

You may well be asked to provide a home care service for someone who has recently come out of hospital. Although a community nurse will normally also be involved for medical care, most of the personal care will be undertaken by the home care service, possibly on a short-term basis, until a full recovery is made, but possibly on a longer-term basis.

You need to be aware that people who are discharged early from hospital may require specialised medical equipment to support them in their own home. You also need to be aware that the pressure on hospital beds can lead to people being discharged too soon – before they are ready – and the rate of readmissions is increasing. You will need to watch out for any signs of deterioration in the person's condition and report it immediately. In such situations the name and number of a contact point should be prominently displayed.

Continuing care is the term which is used to describe the care required by people who do not need to be in hospital for acute medical care, but do have an ongoing need for personal care due to a medical condition from which they are unlikely to recover, for example a severe stroke. The majority of these people will be cared for in their own homes for as long as possible – with the support of home care and the community nursing service. As with short-term recovery care, you need to be alert to signs of deterioration and take the appropriate action.

**In summary** An increasing number of people are discharged early from hospital to recover in their own homes. You will find that you are providing a personal care service (in conjunction with nursing care) in the short term to people who are recovering and in the longer term to people who require continuing care.

# Caring for people who are confused

Confusion may have many causes, but is never due to ageing alone. Treatment may help and even cure the problem. Try to make sure that a cause is sought so that suitable help can be arranged.

Many older people living at home exhibit some degree of confusion. Memory loss, combined with disorientation and wandering, can be very difficult and tiring to deal with. Nevertheless, the aim of any support provided should be to improve the person's quality of life and to seek ways of eliminating or reducing the confusion, if this is possible.

You will require patience and understanding. Many people who are confused live with personal family carers who will need help as well. If they have been caring alone for a confused person for any length of time, they are likely to exhibit signs of stress and to be both physically and mentally exhausted.

There can be many different physical causes of confusion in older people. It should therefore always be assumed that some improvement could be possible.

- With the agreement of the person concerned and their family carer and your line manager, arrange a medical examination if confusion occurs or increases.
- Try to make sense of irrational behaviour.
- Do not label as 'confused' people who may just be forgetful, temporarily disorientated or having difficulty hearing.

Try to understand confused behaviour or speech. Find out about:

- previous medical history, personality and mental state;
- previous social skills and habits, including social isolation, or loss of independence;
- the possible side effects of current medication;
- recent major events such as admission to hospital or a bereavement;
- possible sight or hearing impairment;
- any recurring patterns of abnormal behaviour.

You need to be aware of, and understand, the value and purpose of trying to correct confused ideas.

Correct mistakes gently, without direct contradiction. Distract on to safer topics if necessary; getting the confused person to think of something else may change behaviour that is putting others at risk or causing distress.

'Reality orientation' is the name given to the technique of communicating with a confused person and trying to keep them in touch with reality. Try using these approaches:

- Give frequent reminders of time, place and identity.
- Use the person's name frequently.
- Gently, but firmly, correct confused behaviour, but avoid confrontation.
- Reinforce non-confused behaviour with praise.

To help confused people keep in touch with reality, the following may be of assistance:

- Large clocks or calendars, provided they are kept up to date.
- Well-placed mirrors.

You may also need sensitivity in dealing with neighbours and other family carers, who may have different views on what constitutes appropriate care for the confused person. They may not understand the rights the person has to remain in their own home with all the risks that this entails (see Chapter 2).

**In summary** You can be of great assistance in helping the confused person keep in touch with reality by trying to understand their confused behaviour, gently correcting mistakes and applying the techniques of 'reality orientation'.

# People with challenging behaviour

Unfortunately, physical attacks on staff providing social care are becoming all too common. It may not be the person you are caring for who is aggressive, but a member of their family. You need to be aware of the underlying cause of the aggression, for example is it:

- the consequence of a medical or psychological condition?
- a reaction to a reduction in the level or type of care services being provided?
- a response to your personal actions, manner or speech?

In the first two examples there may be little you can do personally, but in the third you need to understand what you are saying or doing which is leading to an aggressive response and modify your behaviour accordingly.

Training should be available to all Home Carers to:

- increase understanding of the causes of aggression;
- provide information on the way in which potentially violent situations should be handled to defuse the situation and reduce the tension.

You should never go alone in situations where aggression is thought to be likely – two Home Carers should be present. Any attack must be reported to your line manager immediately. If the attack leads to injury – however minor – you must follow the normal accident reporting procedure.

One point is worth making. You are not expected to like everyone simply because they have become old and in need of care. It is not human nature to like and get on with everyone you meet. Although, as mentioned in Chapter 2, many agencies will make every effort to match the personalities of the person needing care and their Home Carer, this is not always possible and you may, on occasions, find yourself providing care to someone you do not really like. This is a natural human reaction. Remember that someone who was difficult to please and bad tempered when young is almost certain to be just the same when they are old – if not worse!

**In summary** Take care to ensure that you do nothing to trigger an aggressive response. If the situation is known to be difficult, two Home Carers should attend together.

# Personal safety of people receiving care

It is not uncommon for Home Carers to be faced with the problem of a person who appears to be acting against their own best interests by putting themselves (and others) at risk in some way.

In Chapter 2 we considered the importance of safeguarding the rights of individuals, including the right to take risks. This includes the right of people receiving care to make decisions and choices which may affect their own health. The dividing line between allowing personal choice and encouraging risk-taking can at times be very fine.

Your employing organisation should have a policy on risk-taking and a system for monitoring and recording risks without necessarily interfering unless the risk is going to become so great that it will affect the health of the person involved.

## Informing on matters of serious concern

You will find that, in time, you as a Home Carer will often know more about the person you are caring for than anyone else. Sometimes you may find yourself in the position of becoming aware of unacceptable or even criminal practices involving the person and undertaken by others including, for example, members of the family, friends, other carers.

This may include:

- physical/sexual abuse;
- mental cruelty;
- theft (money, jewellery, antiques, furniture);
- coercion (to change a Will, enter a residential home, etc).

Your first duty in these circumstances is to protect the person you are caring for. Any practices that may involve any of the above and/or the possibility of risk to the individual concerned must be reported at once to your line manager. This is sometimes known as 'whistleblowing'.

## People who refuse to care for themselves

People you care for may, for example, refuse to take a bath or even wash; live in a dirty and infested house; fill their home with old newspapers; keep many cats – all these situations can happen.

In a recent case an old man starved himself to death, despite almost daily visits from Home Carers and twice-weekly visits from the community nurse. In the end, no one could force him to eat against his will. That was his choice and his decision.

There can be no specific guidelines for coping with these situations, as each set of circumstances will be different. The risks involved in these situations should have been identified at the time the risk assessment was undertaken and appropriate support provided to you by your line manager.

If someone's situation begins to deteriorate, this should be reported to your line manager in order to discuss ways of overcoming the difficulty. Provided there is no unacceptable risk to health or safety, or serious interference with the rights of other people, the situation may have to be accepted. Whatever the outcome, it is important to understand and to remain sympathetic to the needs and wishes of each individual person.

Always remember that the prime responsibility for the mental and physical health of the person rests with the GP, district nurse, community psychiatric nurse or other involved health professional. The role of the Home Carer is to play a part in promoting the health care of the person under medical guidance and, in difficult cases, under medical supervision. A Home Carer is not a nurse, and should not try to act like one.

Please see also ' Standards of cleanliness – pests and infestation' in Chapter 7 (pp 131–133) for further information.

## Abuse of older people

It is now recognised that adults, especially older people, as well as children, may be abused. They could be abused by someone they know – a member of the family or a friend who is looking after them, someone who works in their home or garden, or by strangers who call at their home.

If your employing organisation has a policy on abuse, this should have been covered in your induction. If you are not sure, ask your line manager what you should do if you suspect that the person you are caring for is being abused.

The abuse may take different forms, the most common of which are shown in the table on the following page. It is important to remember that abuse may not be obvious, it can happen initially by accident and build up over time.

Often the person being abused does not understand why it is happening or perhaps does not recognise that they are being abused. They may feel guilt or shame, particularly if they have been sexually abused, and they may not know who to turn to.

| Type of abuse | Example |
| --- | --- |
| Physical abuse | Attacks on the person, which might be anything from rough handling leading to bruising through to injury which might end up in admission to hospital. |
| Psychological abuse | Abusive comments, bullying, 'put downs' or insults which make the person feel worthless and useless. |
| Sexual abuse | Anything from unwanted touching and personal contact through to rape. |
| Financial abuse | Putting a person under pressure to leave money, property, etc, in their Will to someone they would not otherwise have left it to. Also pressuring them to pay for things that they would not otherwise choose to pay for. This can include:<br>• stealing money – including not giving the right change;<br>• talking about personal financial problems so that the older person feels they must help out or leave money in their Will;<br>• keeping control over the older person's cheque book and pension book so that they do not have control over their own money;<br>• getting them to sign agreements to pay for something they don't need;<br>• persuading the person not to buy or do something that they want to do, so that the inheritance is not reduced in any way. |
| Neglect | Person is not eating properly, or is unable to wash or bathe, is left soiled if incontinent, not stimulated or is ignored. |

It can be a fine dividing line between maintaining confidentiality and taking necessary action to maintain the physical and emotional health of the person you are caring for. If in doubt and you have any concerns, it is better to err on the side of safety and report your concern to your line manager – even if the person you are caring for has asked you not to. If in doubt contact the Action on Elder Abuse Response Line (details in Appendix 8).

**In summary** Everyone has the right to live their life in the way they choose, provided that this does not place anyone else – including the Home Carer – at risk. However, you also need to be alert to signs that others are abusing the person you are caring for, either physically, emotionally or financially.

# The need for personal relationships

People of all ages have needs for emotional and sexual expression that are normally met through a wide range of different relationships.

Older people have the same rights as any other citizens to make and maintain friendships and personal relationships without interference or censure. Many will still have access to rewarding relationships and the opportunities, through leisure activities, to make new relationships.

Many people who are housebound, however, experience extreme loneliness and emotional deprivation. They have few, if any, opportunities to express their emotions or make new rewarding relationships. You should be aware of their need for emotional expression. You can show warmth and affection by using touch, such as a pat on the hand or shoulder when appropriate, to indicate to them that they are valued in their own right.

## Sexuality

Contrary to what might be believed, older people do have sexual feelings and can enjoy sex as much as anyone else. Sexual activity is one of life's great pleasures and it is not solely the province of the young, as most Home Carers find out for themselves in the course of their work.

Older people, particularly those living on their own, may have a need to express and find outlets for their feelings. You should not be surprised, therefore, if some people you are caring for wish to talk about sexual matters or if signs of sexual activity are in evidence around the home. You should show tact and discretion in responding, discouraging the person only if their behaviour becomes unacceptable.

Whilst you need to recognise the sexual needs of people, this should never mean that you are expected to put up with or condone unacceptable behaviour or expression. Only you can decide what you personally consider to be unacceptable behaviour.

Your employing organisation should have a written policy on equal opportunities and sexual harassment. Obtain a copy and find out how it relates to your work as a Home Carer. You should receive training on these issues.

Some people may behave inappropriately and without any inhibitions because of learning disabilities or dementia. You should discuss any such difficulties with your line manager. People with learning disabilities may be helped by referral for specialist counselling.

There are a number of specialist organisations that may be able to help and advise younger people with physical disabilities.

General points of guidance:

- Always respect a person's privacy. Knock **and wait** to be invited in before entering bedrooms, bathrooms and other private rooms.
- Don't over-react or be judgemental about what you might find in the home in the way of pornographic material, sex aids, dolls. If they are left on public display, you can politely ask for them to be put away, out of sight. If they are persistently left out, report the matter to your line manager.

- Be careful about the 'signals' you send to the person. Don't joke about sexual matters or make suggestive comments or innuendos – your motives might be misunderstood.
- If you are propositioned in any way, politely and firmly refuse. If it continues in an unacceptable way, inform your line manager.
- If you are subjected to sexual touching, ask the person to stop their unacceptable behaviour and inform your line manager. It is not unknown for female carers either to have to go in twos to the homes of some male users or to have to be replaced by a male carer.
- Be careful how and where you touch people, particularly when providing intimate care.
- If you unexpectedly find someone engaged in a sexual activity – leave quickly and discreetly.
- Don't accept any form of sexual harassment. If it persists, inform your line manager.

If at any stage you feel out of your depth or uncomfortable with the way in which the person expresses their sexual and emotional needs (for example, if pornographic material offends you or if you think it is unlawful), discuss it with your line manager.

Everyone has their own individual and different tolerance to and views of sexual matters and materials. These views should be respected, both for you and the person you are caring for. However, clearly sexual advances cannot be tolerated and should be reported to your line manager, as should any form of sexual harassment. This is an issue that requires sensitive handling in terms of initial response and subsequent management.

**In summary** Use tact and discretion in responding to signs of sexual activity. Never put up with unacceptable sexual behaviour or sexual harassment – report it to your line manager. Be careful what signals you give out. Don't joke about sexual matters or flirt. Your motives may be misunderstood.

# CASE STUDY 1 – PHYSICAL AGGRESSION

**Mrs X** is 64 years old and lives at home with her husband. After suffering a series of strokes Mrs X now has restricted mobility, is unable to talk and experiences dramatic mood swings.

It is felt that the couple have had marital problems in the past and Mrs X is extremely jealous of her husband, particularly when he talks to younger women.

The home care service is provided 3 times a day on 7 days a week. The Assistant helps Mr X to get his wife up, washed, dressed, toileted and fed. In the evening the help is provided to assist Mrs X back to bed.

Mrs X is often violent and the home care manager must ensure that the Home Carer is aware of this. Care is taken not to encourage a violent outburst and the Home Carer is instructed to avoid making herself vulnerable. Mrs X has struck the Home Carer over the head when she bent down to replace the footrests on her wheelchair. The Home Carer has to be careful when assisting Mrs X onto the commode because she is inclined to squeeze the top of the carers arms.

Advice is given to the Home Carer so that she can avoid these attacks. All incidents, actions and advice given are carefully recorded on the case file.

## QUESTIONS

1. As a Home Carer, how would you respond to Mrs X? Identify what you would say and what you would do.

2. Identify what you think Mr X's needs will be.

3. What action would you expect the Home Care Manager to take?

## CASE STUDY 2 – POSSIBLE ABUSE

**Mrs A** was discharged from the orthopaedic ward following a fall at home down a flight of stairs when she sustained a fractured neck of femur. She is 91 years old and lives in a large detached house which she owns with her daughter and son-in-law. She has a grand-daughter with learning difficulties who visits the family home every six weeks and another grand-daughter who is a nurse with whom she has more regular contact. Her daughter, Mrs B, has been providing personal care for her mother for the past three years, as well as attending to all domestic tasks.

As well as two visits daily from the home care service, Mrs A received rehabilitative support from the Hospital at Home team (physiotherapist and occupational therapist). Concerns were aroused when the carers reported bruising and scratching to her face. When questioned, Mrs A was not unduly concerned. No statutory intervention was possible or necessary, but concerns remained regarding:

- Mrs A's increasing dependence on her daughter;
- her daughter's possible isolation, being at home all day;
- her daughter's increasing stress due to her own health problems;
- her daughter's forthright and somewhat aggressive attitude.

A case conference was held with the GP, care manager, health visitor and home care manager present. Both Mrs B and her husband were invited, but refused to attend. It was agreed that although Mrs A now required minimal assistance from the home care service with her personal care, it was essential that home care should be ongoing if only to monitor the situation and to report back any further signs of abuse.

## QUESTIONS

1. What would be the role of the Home Carer in this situation?

2. What would you be looking out for?

3. How could the immediate and extended family be involved?

**CHECKLIST – THE HEALTH OF OLDER PEOPLE**

| Do | Do not |
| --- | --- |
| Maintain strict confidentiality about what you know about a person's medical condition. | Encourage older people to put failing health down to 'just part of getting old' or equate old age with ill health or disabilities. |
| Encourage older people to seek proper medical help. | Treat people as 'medical problems' or illnesses, eg 'diabetics', 'epileptics'. |
| Treat people as individuals with medical conditions. | |
| Encourage a healthy lifestyle. | Assume that older people cannot improve in mental and physical health. |
| Pay attention to the social and emotional needs of the people you care for, as well as their physical needs. | Patronise or 'talk down' to the people you care for. |
| Keep a close watch for symptoms of hypothermia. | Gossip or talk about your own personal problems. |
| Assist people who are confused keep in touch with reality. | Attempt to apply direct heat to the skin (eg a hot water bottle) or move a person if you suspect they are suffering from hypothermia. |
| Report any signs of neglect or physical, psychological or financial abuse. | |
| Recognise the need everyone has for close and intimate personal relationships, in particular those people who are housebound and isolated. | Become involved in administering medication without first seeking the permission of your line manager. |
| | Allow your manner, actions or speech to trigger an aggressive response from the person you are caring for or their personal carer. |
| | Put up with unacceptable behaviour and/or harassment. |

# KEY POINTS

- Ageing is a perfectly natural process but people age at different rates and show different signs of ageing.
- The mental and physical condition of an older person can often improve.
- People should never be described as illnesses (eg 'diabetics'). The emphasis must always be on the person, not their illnesses or disabilities.
- Caring for the person's emotional, psychological and social well-being is as important as meeting their physical needs.
- The Home Carer is the person most likely to notice changes in the physical or mental health of the person they are caring for. These should be reported immediately.
- Watch out for signs of hypothermia and know what action to take.
- Assist with the administration of medication only with the full knowledge of the person's GP, district nurse and your line manager. Involve the local community pharmacist if possible.
- You will increasingly be providing care for people who are discharged early from hospital into their own homes. This may be on a short-term basis for those who will make a full recovery or on a longer-term basis for those who require continuing care.
- You will require endless patience and understanding when caring for people who are confused. Reality orientation – trying to keep them in touch with reality – may assist.
- Never visit on your own any home where there is the potential danger of an aggressive or violent attack. Make sure you are accompanied.
- It is perfectly normal for you not to like all the people you care for. After all, not everyone is nice!
- The prime responsibility for the mental and physical well-being of the person rests with their GP and district nurse.
- Home Carers should be aware of the need that people have, in particular those who are housebound, for emotional expression.
- Older people can enjoy sex just as much as younger people.

# 5 Making the First Contact

**S/NVQ Level 2: This chapter relates to the mandatory units O1, CL1 and Z1; Option Group A units CU5, W2; Option Group B units W8, Y1.**

First impressions are always important and never more so than when someone is going to allow you into their own home to undertake personal and practical tasks for them that they were previously able to do for themselves. The first contact requires sensitivity, tact and caution.

All of what follows in this and in subsequent chapters must be considered in the context of the policies and practices of your employing organisation. A list of issues and topics upon which your organisation should have written guidance for your information is included in Appendix 4 of this book. If you have never been provided with this information – ask for it. You need it!

Although you are generally working on your own, you should not be expected to work in a vacuum.

If you are self-employed you might like to think through these issues for yourself and, using *CareFully* as a guide, decide your own policies on these issues. This will then provide a consistent framework for your work with different people with different care needs.

**Remember** – the first impressions are crucial. You are not only representing your organisation, but for most people receiving care you will be the human face of the organisation.

# The importance of the role of the Home Carer

It is recognised that Home Carers have a crucial part to play in the lives of people requiring care and their family and friends. Home Carers are the ones most likely to be in frequent, regular contact with the person they are caring for. They may often become what is known as the 'keyworker' (see p 94), that is the main channel of contact and communication between the person receiving care, any designated 'care manager' they may have (responsible for assessing care needs and developing the care plan) and the organisation or agency commissioned or contracted to provide the care services. A three-way 'contract' is undertaken by all those involved. This is illustrated in the following diagram:

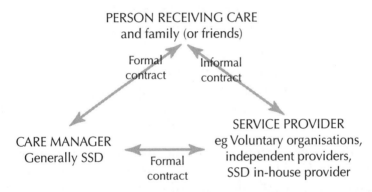

Before undertaking any work as a Home Carer, you should have received the necessary induction training which must include health and safety and moving and lifting. If you are asked to provide any form of specialised care such as operate hoists, administer medication, care of people from ethnic minority communities or people who are terminally ill, you should not be expected to enter the home without the necessary training.

Twenty years ago, the main argument against introducing training for Home Carers was that 'they are only doing in someone else's home what they would do in their own'. Today we recognise that that is not true. Every home, person and situation is different and all Home Carers need training in order to respond appropriately to individual needs.

**In summary**  The Home Carer has the key role in terms of regular contact with the person needing care.

# Before starting work in the home

Before starting work in someone's home you should have basic information about that person and their care needs. This may be extracted from their personal care plan or care assessment. Basic information includes their general level of physical ability, mobility, any special health, religious or cultural requirements and information on the actual caring tasks you are required to do. You should also be provided with information on the risk assessment that was undertaken so that you are aware from the outset of any particular risks that are attached to providing the care. If you do not have this basic information, ask your employing organisation for it.

You should also be informed of the standards to which you are expected to work and any quality assurance measures which are to be applied to ensure that you are meeting the standards. These need to be taken into account when discussing the standard required by the person you are caring for – see the next section.

Your employing organisation should also identify and inform you of tasks you should not undertake. These are generally because they represent a health and safety hazard to you, and/or the person you are caring for (see Chapter 7, 'Health and Safety'). The sorts of tasks involved include lifting heavy objects, moving heavy furniture, any activity that involves standing on ladders, etc. If in doubt, ask your agency or employing organisation. You also need to be aware of tasks you are not required to undertake because they have not been assessed as a priority activity upon which you should spend your time and an element of public money.

## Involvement of other agencies in the care plan

You also need to know who else and what other agencies are also providing care services to that person. You may need to coordinate with them and schedule your visits to fit in with and meet the needs of the person you are caring for and their family carers. For example, it is not sensible for you to arrive at the same time that the district or community nurse comes to give the person a bath or change dressings and the 'meals on wheels' are delivered. Besides the problem of everything happening at once, it does not help to break up the day for someone who may be housebound.

This is particularly important if the person is living alone and is confined to home. It will help reduce isolation if all those involved in providing care can visit on different days or at different times of the day. There is no point in everyone arriving at once. You will only get in one another's way and it will not help the person you are caring for.

## Provision of information

You also need to be aware of what information the person has received. Do they have a copy of their own care plan? Do they have some form of contract or agreement with your employing organisation? What are their expectations of you and what you are going to do? Do they know what their rights are? Are they aware of the complaints procedure? Have any unmet needs been recorded and, if so, where?

The survey of people receiving home care mentioned on page 66 found that the majority of the people interviewed had very little information in writing – or if they had it had been mislaid. Key information on the care plan, name and telephone number of persons to contact in an emergency, organisation providing care, care manager and the complaints procedure should always be kept in a safe place.

There is a lot of basic information you require right from the start.

**In summary** Ensure you have all the essential information you require, concerning the service you will provide, before starting work in the home.

# The Home Carer as the 'keyworker'

As a Home Carer you will be the one person (other than relatives or friends) who will be in the most frequent and regular contact with the person requiring care. You will inevitably build up a relationship. This role is sometimes called that of keyworker. You are therefore in the best position to judge if those care needs have changed, if the situation and circumstances have altered and if further help and support are required.

Any such changes should always be reported to your line manager and/or employing organisation to enable them to take appropriate action, including a 'reassessment' of the care needs. However tempting it is to do 'that bit extra' for the person you are caring for, you should never try to meet the further needs yourself without the agreement of your employer, because that could be breaking the terms of the contract between the social services department 'purchasing' care from your employing organisation. You may also find that in certain circumstances (eg climbing ladders) it cancels any occupational insurance under which you are covered by your employer.

## 'Matching' people needing care and Home Carers

It is a sign of the importance of the Home Carer's role that many employing organisations try to 'match', as far as possible, the needs and personality of the person requiring care with those of the Home Carer. It is becoming increasingly common for employing agencies to invite people needing care, and any family or personal carer they may have, to choose between two or three possible Home Carers. This is consistent with the desire to involve people receiving care in decisions relating to that care and to maximise their choice wherever possible.

You should not be surprised, nor upset or offended, if you are not 'chosen' to be someone's Home Carer, provided you have not been discriminated against. There is absolutely no point in inflicting contrasting personalities on one another, or you may be physically unsuited for the personal care tasks required. It is essential that the person receiving care and any family carer involved feel relaxed, secure and comfortable with the Home Carer they have chosen.

Unfortunately there are two related factors which make it difficult in certain circumstances to provide a choice in who provides the home care.

Firstly, a change in the profile of the population makes it difficult to recruit Home Carers, particularly in certain parts of the country. Put simply, we have an ageing population and there are fewer people available for the work, particularly in areas of relatively high employment. This in itself makes it difficult to provide choice.

Secondly, there is an increase in the level of dependency and complexity of care needs of people who are now staying in their own homes, where before 1993 they would have gone into residential homes. It is therefore becoming common for 'teams' of Home Carers to be allocated to provide care to the same person – either in pairs, to assist with moving and lifting, for example when getting the person in and out of bed, or to provide care at different times of day and seven days a week. Whereas it may be possible to allow choice if there is only one, or even two Home Carers involved, it becomes almost impossible if there are three or four.

## Caring for people from ethnic minority communities

In order to ensure that people needing care who belong to ethnic minority communities get the same services as others, special attention should be paid to the following points.

### LANGUAGE

For many people from ethnic minority communities, English is not their first language. Never assume an understanding of what a person may be saying; for example, someone being 'difficult' about eating their food may be trying to indicate that the food is contrary to their religion or that they are diabetic. Older people from ethnic minority communities may not understand English. If you find yourself working in this situation, it would show sensitivity to try to learn a few key words in the relevant language.

Has the person needing care been given information, for example the care plan or the complaints procedure, in their own language? If not, how much are they really able to understand about the process, what they are entitled to, what you are able to help with, etc? How confusing do you think it is, not to have information in your own language? Is there any way you think this could be overcome?

**Interpreters**

Whenever difficulties occur, and always for the first meeting, an interpreter should be used. (It is not permissible to use children for this.) Some areas have an interpreting service, or the local community relations council may help.

## CULTURE

You need to understand about significant religious days; for example, Diwali (Festival of Light) is important to Sikhs and Hindus, and Ramadan to Muslims, just as Easter is to Christians.

## SERVICE PROVISION

Whenever appropriate and possible, Home Carers should be recruited from within the same ethnic community as the person needing care. Unfortunately, this is not always possible. You may therefore need to be aware of particular needs; for example, Muslims always wash plates and crockery under running water to avoid contamination.

## PROVISION OF FOOD

Particular note should be taken of religious and cultural preferences so that the appropriate diet is observed. In cultures where it is normal to eat with the fingers, the usual feeding aids and utensils will not be required.

## CLOTHES

You will need to know how to assist people with the clothes of their choice and understand what is correct for the occasion and time of day. The local community relations council or religious centre (for example the local temple) can offer advice. You need also to ensure that the clothes you wear will not give offence – for example, sleeveless tops, short miniskirts, low-cut necks – although these are generally unsuitable for working as a Home Carer anyway.

**In summary** You will become the 'keyworker' to the person you are caring for – identifying when needs change and if necessary triggering a reassessment. Wherever possible, effort should be taken to 'match' Home Carers to the people needing care.

# The first working day

It follows from what has already been written that your first entry into the home of the person you are going to care for should be planned and structured. The initial stage of contact is absolutely crucial because the success or otherwise of the first meetings will set the tone for the future of the relationship.

You should not just turn up one morning and start work, hoping that everything will be all right. However, regrettably, this does happen and it is to the credit of both the Home Carer and the person being cared for that, in most cases, the arrangement works.

The process that should be followed is identified in the checklist on page 99. It is often difficult, for many administrative and organisational reasons, for employing organisations to implement this process fully, but they should work towards it.

## *Policy on key-holding*

If the person you are caring for has difficulty getting to the front door, as a regular visitor, they may be pleased to let you have a key to let yourself in. If this is the case you should always:

- Obtain the agreement that you should hold a key in writing from the person you are caring for.
- When not in use, keep the key in a safe place agreed by and known to your line manager as well as the person you are caring for.
- Label the key with a code – never the name and address.

Some organisations providing home care advise the people they are caring for of alternatives, such as the 'Keysafe' home key boxes which enable those who know the combination to obtain the key and enter the home. This avoids the need for the Home Carer to carry a key or the necessity to 'hide' the key somewhere outside the home – a practice which should always be discouraged.

It is courteous to knock or ring the bell before using the key. You could agree a special knock or ring so that the person knows that it is you.

You should also show your identification – at least until the person gets to know you well.

## Whose standards?

You should always be very aware that you are working in someone else's home – not your own – and treat it accordingly.

The tasks you do should have been agreed and clarified in advance between the person needing care, their personal or family carer, and the person putting together the care plan or the care package. If, when you arrive, you find that there is any difference in opinion or expectation about the work you will do, this should be reported immediately to your line manager, who may be in a position to advise who could undertake those tasks that you are either not allowed or not required to do yourself.

However, you should take care to establish from the very beginning exactly how each person wishes you to undertake each task and their personal preferences.

Whose standards should apply? Yours, or those relating to the person receiving care? Very few people have exactly the same standards and you must be open-minded and flexible. Above all, you should never try to impose your standards on others. What is considered a nice, tidy, comfortable home to one person may be a cold, unfriendly and impersonal place to another or a hopeless muddle to a third.

**CHECKLIST – THE PROCESS OF INTRODUCING THE HOME CARER TO THE PERSON NEEDING CARE AND THEIR FAMILY**

- The Home Carer receives appropriate training and preparation before commencing work.
- The decision to provide care is taken following the assessment of care need, sometimes by staff from more than one agency (multi-disciplinary assessment).
- The person needing care should, wherever possible, be able to choose who becomes their Home Carer.
- The Home Carer should have access to the assessment of the care that is required and/or the care plan, and know and understand and be able to discuss its objectives.
- The Home Carer should be introduced to the person requiring care and their family and friends by someone from the agency with whom the person requiring care is familiar.
- The Home Carer should be provided with some form of personal identification by their employing organisation.
- Care should be taken to ensure that everyone involved is completely clear about the role of the Home Carer, the work and activities they will undertake and the level of personal care they will provide.
- The frequency with which the care will be provided must be known to all concerned, but it is sensible to retain a degree of flexibility to allow for sickness, holidays or other unforeseen events.
- Substitute arrangements to provide care in the Home Carer's absence should be discussed and agreed in principle with all concerned.
- Measures for monitoring the quality of care provided and maintaining standards should be agreed by all concerned.
- There should be regular reviews of the care programme (or care package) at agreed times, to ensure that the care provided continues to meet the person's needs. The Home Carer and the service user and family carers must be involved in the review. *Modernising Social Services* proposes the first review is undertaken after three months and at least annually thereafter.
- All concerned need to understand that, in spite of making every effort to give the person and their carers choice in the services that are provided, and listening to their views, there may be occasions when what the individual and the family want may not be what the caring agency can provide, nor what it thinks is appropriate.

Your aim is to enable each individual person to lead as normal a life as possible within their normal surroundings. You therefore, within reason, assume their standards. However, this will have to be balanced against the standards required by the organisation you work for. If there is a significant gap between the two, you should discuss it with your line manager.

This does not necessarily mean that you cannot make certain changes such as moving furniture, washing crockery, throwing away papers and food, etc, but only with the complete permission of the person you are caring for.

Hygiene standards can also be an area of concern. This is an issue that is picked up in Chapter 7, 'Health and Safety'.

 How would you describe your own personal standards? How do you think that these may relate to or affect the people you are caring for? How do you think you really feel about other people's standards?

## Matching wants, needs and the provision of services

In spite of taking every effort in the early stages to clarify expectations and to involve the person being cared for and their family in all the decisions relating to the care, misunderstandings and differences of opinion do and will occur. Two examples will illustrate the point:

1 A person with care needs and their family place a high value on the cleanliness of the home. This is an important consideration, particularly where the person has been very houseproud. The care team/agency, although accepting the need for minimum standards of cleanliness, places the emphasis on the use of scarce home care time in providing physical care and in ensuring that vital shopping is done and money matters are dealt with. Whilst a compromise may be necessary, it is not always easy to achieve.

2 The need may be to provide care at times that are not covered by a personal family carer; for example, early mornings, late

evenings, weekends (known as 'unsocial hours'). Although more flexible schemes have been developed over recent years to meet these needs, it is not always possible to meet the exact requirements of the person and their family in this respect.

 **Can you think of other examples of differences of opinion and views between professionals, agencies providing care and the person receiving care and their family?**

**What was the outcome? Do you think that it was the right one in the circumstances?**

These examples illustrate that you may sometimes find yourself working to two service users – the person with care needs and their personal family carer. You will need to discuss and clarify with both (separately and/or together) the tasks they are expecting to be done, how and in what order. It is not unknown for differences of opinion and even conflict to arise, and you may need considerable negotiating and mediating skills to reach agreement on exactly what both parties are expecting you to do.

**In summary** Your first introduction into the home should be carefully planned wherever possible. You should be aware of the particular wants, needs and standards of the people you are caring for and meet these needs as appropriate. Ensure that keys to the home are kept in a safe place.

## Sources of assistance

As well as the help that can be expected from your own agency, it is also good practice to draw up a list together with the person you are caring for and their family and friends, of other sources of help, such as those identified in the following checklist. This should be done when you first begin work with a new person receiving services.

Not all the information will be either available or required but you should be able to obtain the essential details.

This list should be kept in a prominent place, with the agreement of the person concerned, for ease of reference; for example, by the telephone or by the front or back door.

It is very easy with modern computer equipment for your care agency to provide you and all your colleague Home Carers with a printed list that could be filled in. If you do not have one already, why not suggest it to them? The list should also be available in the appropriate format for the individual person; for example, in the language generally used by that person or in large type or braille for people who are partially sighted.

Very often the actual existence and details of such sources of assistance can help the person needing care and their family to feel more secure – not to mention the Home Carer!

You will also need to be aware of national and local voluntary organisations that provide services and/or equipment. The list of organisations and their addresses in Appendix 8 is a starting point.

**In summary** The principal sources of assistance are summarised in the following checklist.

**SOURCES OF HELP**

| | Name | Address | Telephone number |
|---|---|---|---|
| Family | | | |
| Friends | | | |
| GP | | | |
| Care Manager | | | |
| Home Carer | | | |
| Home Care Agency | | | |
| District Nurse | | | |
| Pharmacist | | | |
| Dentist | | | |
| Chiropodist | | | |
| Hairdresser | | | |
| Housing Department or Landlord | | | |
| Religious Leader | | | |
| Welfare Rights | | | |
| Social Services | | | |
| Social Security | | | |
| Solicitor | | | |
| Local Age Concern Group | | | |
| Voluntary Organisations | | | |

# CASE STUDY

## The A Family

Two years ago, the home care service were asked to provide personal care/support to three profoundly handicapped children of a Muslim family. The family has an average of 70 hours care a week, originally being provided by an agency specialising in children with learning disabilities. The agency was unable to sustain this level of care and the home care service were asked to share the care.

Besides the normal problems involved introducing a new team into the family, there was the greater problem of the staff understanding the different cultural needs.

Hygiene is extremely important to Muslims. It is important that males and females are segregated and since there are two girls and one boy, all the clothing must be kept separate, even to the extent of collecting soiled linen and washing it separately. A separate bath mat must be used for the girls. All bedding must be changed every day and each child must have their own bed linen, towel, flannel, toothbrush, toothpaste and hairbrush.

The children must be washed in running water at all times and after going to the toilet they must have their hands washed in running water with a separate bar of soap. When bathing under running water, under no circumstances must the flannel touch the side of the bath and the towel must not touch the floor, even though there is a clean incontinent sheet put on the floor for each child. The bath has to be disinfected after each child's use.

All three children are profoundly handicapped but the boy is the most severely handicapped. His mother insisted that the home care staff walked him to the car, although he isn't capable of walking and was more or less lifted to the car in which he travelled for day care. This car was an ordinary taxi and it was impossible to get him in properly. Also some of the taxi drivers were less than sympathetic. A case conference was called and reluctantly the mother agreed to try taking him in a wheelchair so the boy could sit in comfort on his journey. This has proved very successful and the mother agrees that it was the best for all concerned.

The family are very hospitable and little plates of sweetmeats are offered and small gifts of food given, which although may not be to the Home Carer's taste, must be accepted as it would offend to refuse.

The home care service has since taken on the grandfather of these children, who lives nearby, and a similar cultural requirement of washing in running water has to be followed. His hair has to be washed three times and his face twice.

When the Home Carers first took over his care they were not allowed to wash his genitals, his wife had to do this and she had to be present at all times of personal care. This has now been changed and his wife accepts the Home Carers and leaves them to get on with their job.

In the beginning, there were quite a few problems but now the care packages are working well.

## QUESTIONS

1. How do you think you would feel working in this environment?

2. What training do you think you would require?

3. What basic care needs do you think the children have in addition to their cultural and religious needs?

# KEY POINTS

■ The Home Carer is of vital importance in the life of the person being cared for, as the person most frequently in regular contact (the keyworker).

■ Whenever possible, people needing care should be involved in decisions on who becomes their Home Carer, and given a choice.

■ The Home Carer must have detailed information of the care plan or the assessed need and know who else is involved in providing care.

■ The initial introduction of the Home Carer into the home must be planned and structured.

■ It is important to involve service users and their family carers in decisions relating to their care, and enable them to contribute to the care plan and clarify expectations.

■ The Home Carer must always respond with sensitivity and understanding to the needs of the person they are caring for – including their cultural and religious needs – and separately to the particular needs of the family carer.

■ Employing organisations and agencies must provide Home Carers with support and basic information on policies and practices, in order to enable them to provide a high-quality service. This cannot be achieved when working in a vacuum.

■ A list of key telephone numbers should be kept in a prominent place in the home of each person receiving care.

# 6

# The Basic Skills of Home Carers

**S/NVQ Level 2: This chapter relates to the mandatory units O1, CL1 CU1 and Z1; Option Group A units CU5, W2; Option Group B units CU3, W8, Y1.**

This chapter explores the issues involved in starting to work in someone else's home. It looks at whose standards should be applied and goes on to discuss some of the basic activities that the Home Carer undertakes. In order to avoid repetition, some activities are covered more fully in subsequent chapters (for example providing meals and helping with eating and drinking).

## Arriving at the home

Please always try to be on time. People who receive care appreciate their Home Carers being punctual, reliable and dependable.

You should always knock on the door, even if you have a key to the home. It is probably also sensible to either agree a special knock or ring or to call out so that the person you are visiting knows who it is. It is also good practice on arrival to show your identity card, although realistically once you become known to the person you are caring for, this is unlikely to continue to be necessary.

You must always remember that when you enter the home of a person who needs care, you do so at their invitation – an invitation that they have the right to withdraw at any time. There is absolutely no obligation on anyone at any time to accept a service that they may very well need, but which they do not want.

Some organisations issue Home Carers with monitoring devices such as swipe cards or pens. If you have one of these, you may need to use it to record the time of your arrival in the home. As the volume of home care provided by private and voluntary sector agencies on behalf of local authority social services departments increases, so there is likely to be a corresponding increase in the use of these devices.

Also on arrival at the home, you should check with the person you are caring for whether there is anything in particular that needs to be done. Although the activities and tasks you undertake will be part of the care plan, there should be sufficient flexibility to vary the routine slightly on occasions. However, this should not become a regular occurrence. If it does, it indicates either that a reassessment of care needs is required, or that the person is trying to get more work done that is not considered a priority for you to do.

If the person receives a complex package of care including (for example) regular visits from the district or community nurse and meals on wheels, and there is a mechanism for recording these visits in a log, you should always check to see who has visited and whether they left any note or comment. This could be important as it may indicate something that you need to pick up in your work, or refer back to your line manager.

If no such log is available, but you think it would be useful, you might like to suggest it to your line manager.

**In summary**  Knock or ring the doorbell before entering. Check any record or notes that may have been left by a district nurse, etc. Activate any monitoring devices and ask the person what they would like to be done.

## Starting work

The home and all its possessions must always be treated with respect and objects handled with care. Accidents can and will happen, as everyone recognises, but care should be taken to prevent them occurring, if at all possible. If the person you are caring for has poor vision and is unable to see clearly, avoid moving objects and furniture from their usual place, where the person will be used to finding them.

Unless asked to find a personal document or possession, you should never look through private papers or personal belongings.

When in someone else's home you should never make yourself a cup of tea or coffee, help yourself to biscuits, etc, unless you are invited to do so. Remember at all times that you are not in your own home, but in someone else's.

If you smoke, it is good practice not to do so in someone else's home, even if they smoke themselves. Wait until you are out of the home and moving on to your next visit. Many employers do not allow their Home Carers to smoke while on duty. Even if it is not a policy of your particular agency, it is always good practice not to smoke.

Some people you care for may be heavy smokers. If this causes you any difficulty as their carer, please talk to your line manager about it.

Above all, you should always remember that you are there to assist the person remain in their own home. This means supporting and maintaining their independence as far as possible. You should there-fore always encourage the people to do as much as possible for themselves and never automatically do things for them that they could do for themselves – unless there is a very good reason why you should do it.

Agree on certain tasks that can be left for the person to carry out themselves, taking into account their degree of disability. Encourage them to undertake tasks with you if possible and involve them in the running of the home. Always avoid increasing their dependence. Remember the phrase 'use it or lose it' – it particularly applies to maintaining someone's independence.

**In summary** Show respect for the person's possessions and their right to privacy. Do not smoke while on duty and do not help yourself to tea, coffee or biscuits without being invited to do so. Encourage the person you are caring for to do as much as possible for themselves in order to maintain their independence.

# Health and safety

You must always take account of health and safety in your work – both your health and safety and that of the person you are caring for. All employing organisations must have policies relating to health and safety as a result of the Health and Safety at Work etc Act 1974 (HASAWA), which is now amended by the European Directive on Manual Handling (90/269/EEC). Information on these policies should be part of your induction training.

Check up on the policies and find out what you can and cannot do. Most organisations have some regulations relating to (for example) not climbing ladders.

An assessment of the risks involved in providing care in the home will have been undertaken by either your line manager or a designated manager in your organisation. You should be fully aware of any risks associated with the work you undertake, before you begin work. These risks will cover the physical condition of the home, the physical condition of the furniture and equipment in the home and any hazards associated with the work you do, including manual handling and pets!

Remember that you should never be expected to lift heavy or awkward loads – and this includes people. You can all too easily strain your back and have to take time off work, which will be neither good for you nor the people you care for. Never agree to lift heavy loads, even as a favour. It will not do you any good in the long run.

In some homes factors such as poor lighting, cluttered furniture and worn or frayed carpets can represent safety hazards to the person living in the home and everyone who visits it. In these situations you can only advise the person or their family to make changes and try gentle persuasion. If you are seriously concerned about a hazard, report it to your line manager.

## Hygiene practice

Hygiene is also part of health and safety and can be quite a problem in the provision of home care services, as standards can vary so considerably. You need to take all necessary precautions to prevent the risk of infection, not only to yourself but also to ensure that you do not transfer any infection and or infestation from one home to another that you visit.

This means that you must regularly wash your hands and dry them thoroughly. It is the single most important action you can take to reduce the spread of infection. If you have any form of cut or graze on your hand, this should be covered by a waterproof dressing which is regularly replaced.

All employers should provide some form of protective clothing to wear while working. This will include protective gloves and aprons and/or overalls which should always be worn when there is the slightest chance of infection and when undertaking personal care tasks when you may come into contact with body fluids. Protection may also be provided for your head and hair and for your feet.

Many people you are caring for may not like you wearing the protective clothing. You will need to be sensitive to this and explain that it is for their own protection as well as yours and the others you are caring for.

More information on health and safety may be found in Chapter 7.

**In summary** You have a duty to yourself, the people you are caring for and your employing organisation to adopt safe working practices at all times and to take all the precautions necessary to avoid the risk of spreading infection and infestation.

# Basic care activities

As a Home Carer, you will be required to carry out a number of important and often personal or intimate services for the person you are caring for.

The following guidance describes the principal basic care activities which should always be undertaken, with good humour, sensitivity to the needs and feelings of the person receiving the care and flexibility.

Further information on some of these tasks may be found in the relevant chapters of this book.

## Helping people to get out of bed

If one of your tasks is to help people to get up, make certain that any routine is flexible; some older people will wish to get up immediately upon waking; others will need time to prepare themselves. Where possible, the time of each morning visit should take into account the wishes and preferences of the person you are assisting.

**Always** knock before entering the room, and wait to be invited in – don't walk in at the same time as you knock! Open the door slowly so as not to startle the person. This is particularly important if they have difficulty hearing and may not have heard your knock.

Ask if they are ready to get up. If they are not, and there is no urgent reason for them to do so, attend to other tasks until they wish to get up. However, the gap between the first greeting and returning to assist with getting up should not be longer than about a quarter of an hour, particularly where attempts to get out of bed unaided could lead to a fall.

Talk to the person about the day ahead and what they are going to do in a way that is relevant to them, bearing in mind their circumstances and lifestyle.

Assist the person to the toilet or commode if necessary.

Keep alert for any signs of incontinence, illness or injury, such as difficulty with breathing, coughing, bruising, weakness of upper limbs, numbness. Always enquire very sensitively about any such signs in order not to alarm the person you are caring for.

Many older people receiving home care now receive assistance with the personal care tasks associated with getting up and going to bed but may not receive any other assistance from the service during the day. Unfortunately this can lead to very short visits – 15 to 20 minutes have been known. You may therefore be very pressured in terms of fitting everything in to the time available, with insufficient time to talk to the person you are caring for, to be sensitive and able to respond to any particular needs they may have. You need to be very aware of the pressure and stress this may place on the person you are caring for, in particular if they move slowly and/or need to take their time getting up or going to bed. If you think the pattern of service delivery is causing any distress, do report it to your line manager.

## Dressing and undressing

**Always** respect the person's privacy and dignity. There is no need to stay in the room if the person is able to dress or partially dress themselves. You should encourage as much independence in dressing and undressing as possible.

Always let the person choose for themselves what they wish to wear – it enhances their self-esteem. However, you may need to assist someone with poor sight or visual disability to match colours.

You need to be conscious of, and sensitive to, the frustration that can be generated by weakness and loss of ability. Offer help sympathetically; allow plenty of time and don't rush, taking into account any illness, physical impairment or disability. A positive attitude is more likely to encourage an interest in personal appearance.

You will need to know exactly what help each person needs and that a particular method of dressing might be necessary; for example, someone who has suffered a stroke might be unaware of their affected side. Simple aids may also assist the person to dress themselves (for example, something to help pull up a zip on the back of a dress). The advice of the occupational therapist can always be sought to help you help the people you are caring for.

Some people may find it easier to dress themselves if clothes are laid out. Clothes should be selected in advance to ensure that a person is never left undressed while a new set of clothes is sought.

## Washing, shaving and dental care

Most people wish to continue to look after their personal hygiene themselves for as long as possible and you should do everything to encourage this.

Some people may be becoming forgetful or unaware of the need for concern for their personal hygiene. In these circumstances you may need to tactfully remind them and you may have to assist with the everyday tasks of washing, shaving and looking after their hair and teeth.

For most people, their self-respect is enhanced when they feel clean and comfortable. There should be emphasis on:

- Regular washing of hands and face.
- Regular combing of hair.
- For men without a beard, regular shaving at a frequency best suited to the needs of the individual (an electric razor may allow them to do it for themselves).
- Regular cleaning of teeth or dentures.
- Cleaning of spectacles.

**Note** The cutting or trimming of either finger or toenails should always be carried out by an appropriately qualified person or by a district nurse or chiropodist. Don't try to do it yourself – particularly if you do not have the qualifications. If you accidentally cut or nick a person, this can cause infection and other complications, particularly if they are diabetic. Some voluntary organisations, including some local Age Concern groups, will trim nails.

## Bathing

Whenever possible, people should be encouraged to bath themselves. However, they may feel more secure taking a bath when someone else is in the home, in case anything goes wrong or they fall. Or they may wish assistance in and out of the bath, particularly if it has high sides.

The occupational therapist may be able to advise on the installation of handles to grip or steps to assist getting in and out of the bath. Other bath aids include a rubber mat to prevent slipping in the bath and special grips to turn the handles of the taps.

The installation of an independent shower unit and cabinet can assist people who are not as agile as they once were, or with mobility difficulties. However, this can be relatively expensive and many older people in particular prefer to have a bath.

Taking a bath does not have to be a regular routine, and a person's preference in this matter is likely to be determined by the habits of a lifetime. The time of a bath should be arranged taking this into consideration. Bathing should be a pleasant experience which is enjoyed.

Wherever possible, assistance with bathing should always be carried out by the regular carer who is most familiar and comfortable with the person having the bath. Always check the temperature of the water before allowing the person to use the bath. Dipping the elbow in is the traditional and easy way of doing this.

Always allow the person time for a relaxing and therapeutic soak if they wish to do so. Check for any obvious signs of illness, bruising or disability, sensitively. If possible, leave the person alone in the bathroom for a while, if necessary remaining within earshot in case help is needed.

In accordance with lifting and handling regulations (see p 138), if the person actually requires lifting into or out of the bath, equipment such as a hoist should be made available. Never try to lift the person yourself, even if there are two of you. You could hurt the person you are assisting, as well as damage yourself. Many older people are reluctant to use the hoist, nevertheless you should reassure them that it is for their own personal safety as well as yours

If you need to assist by providing a steady hand and support, be sensitive to the intimacy of the situation and recognise that the person may be embarrassed. Remember their rights to privacy, dignity and respect, identified in Chapter 2.

As an alternative to a bath, encourage the person to take a shower or have a strip wash. They may be able to do this unaided.

Sometimes some people forget to wash or bathe and may not recognise that they need to do so for hygienic reasons. A simple but tactful reminder may be enough.

Refusal to bathe may be for various sensitive reasons such as embarrassment that physical help is needed and they can't do it for themselves, the threat of being touched, shame about incontinence, or the desire to hide the evidence of incontinence. If you suspect that this is the case, seek advice from your line manager.

## Medication

You may be asked by the person you are caring for, their GP or the District Nurse to assist with administering medication. Any such requests should always be reported to your line manager and their permission obtained in writing. There is more on medication in Chapter 4, 'The Health of Older People'.

## Assisting with meals

Eating can be one of life's pleasures, and a social activity. Meal times should be looked forward to, and time should be spent with people while they eat.

When shopping, make sure some foods that require no preparation, such as bread, cheese, cold meats, fruit and breakfast cereals, are bought so that the person you are caring for can get their own meals with ease.

If one of your tasks is to prepare a person's meal – breakfast, lunch or supper – where possible, it should be provided at a time which suits that person, encouraging them to choose the menu and have a balanced diet, including plenty of fruit and vegetables.

Ensure that you observe the rules of hygiene. Always take care when handling food. Remember to wash your hands before touching food and to use clean containers and utensils. Dispose of any food in the kitchen which is past its 'use by' date or not as fresh as it should be, with the permission of the person you are caring for.

Care should be taken to lay the table or tray attractively, ensuring that food looks appetising on the plate. If the person is confused, it may be necessary to watch and if necessary to assist to ensure that they eat the meal you have prepared.

Always allow plenty of time for eating meals and avoid rushing. Further information may be found in Chapter 8, 'Eating and Nutrition'.

## Shopping

If shopping is undertaken, it is important to remember to encourage the person's independence and participation in the process.

If at all possible, take the person with you. This not only gives the individual the chance to get out of the house but also enables them to choose the items they want and to see what else is available.

If the person has a sight problem, you should ask them how they would like you to escort them. Some people may prefer to take your arm, in which case you should walk slightly ahead of them and indicate when you get to kerbs. In shops you will need to read out labels and prices and – most helpfully – spot the special offers!

If it is not possible to take the person with you, try to involve them in preparing and preferably writing a detailed shopping list, which identifies not only what they want but also where it should be bought – if possible.

When handling cash or cheques, it is important to go through it clearly with the individual; for example, 'I have taken a £10 note out of your purse for the shopping today'. It is important to keep a written record of all financial transactions which can be easily referred to if a query arises. Always obtain a receipt for any goods purchased so that you can account for any money spent. This is covered in more detail in Chapter 11, 'Financial Matters'.

An awareness of the problems older people face when trying to eat healthily is necessary; it may be important on occasions to be able to give advice on budgeting for healthy eating. This is followed up in Chapter 8.

When putting the shopping away, ensure that food is stored correctly, and always in accordance with the instructions on the packaging. Most people with poor sight will have their own system for keeping certain types of food in particular places. If possible, the person should put the food away themselves as you read out the labels. This will help them find it again.

Remember that medicines and household cleaning agents that you have bought are potentially dangerous; care should therefore be taken with the storage, handling and disposal of such items. Again this is particularly important for people with poor sight. Medicines must be clearly identifiable. This may be done by using a special shape of container or labelling in large print or braille.

## Going to bed

If you are responsible for helping to get someone to bed, remember that everyone likes to go to bed when it suits them. They may have long-established bed-time routines, which must be respected.

- Establish exactly what help is needed at bed-time.
- Avoid hustling and hurrying.
- Be prepared to be patient.
- As already identified, many people will be able to look after their own personal hygiene, but they may need some encouragement. Use good humour and gentle persuasion.
- If the person you are caring for does need help with their personal hygiene, remember to protect their dignity and self-respect at all times.
- If you are providing care for someone who is suffering from incontinence, it is imperative to ensure that good clean skincare practices are followed, regularly washing your hands with soap.
- Be particularly sensitive to any action that might cause embarrassment.
- Seek ways of involving the person you are caring for and gaining their cooperation in whatever care and support must be provided.
- Maintain the person's privacy at all times.

**In summary** Always undertake any care tasks, particularly personal care, with sensitivity and concern for the person you are caring for. Encourage them to be aware of the need for personal hygiene.

# Leaving the home

Check at the end of each visit that tasks have been carried out satisfactorily. If your organisation uses any form of monitoring equipment such as swipe cards or pens or computers, you will need to activate them to record the tasks you have completed and the time you leave the home.

If there is any form of written log kept in the home, that will also need to be brought up to date following your visit.

When leaving the home, ensure that the person is comfortable and that everything necessary is within easy reach; for example, a drink, medication, newspapers, access to the commode.

However, if the person is confused, it may be necessary to ensure that any potential sources of danger are not too accessible – put away medication, check that the cooker and other appliances are switched off, etc.

Make sure that the home is secure and that any external door other than the one you will be leaving by, is locked. If leaving during the day, check that the person knows which windows are open (if any) and that they or someone else will be able to close them at the end of the day. It may be necessary to leave some lights on if the person is not very mobile and there will be no further visitors before it begins to get dark.

Close the door securely, locking any locks necessary.

**In summary** Check that the person concerned is comfortable and the house is secure before you leave. Bring any recording systems up to date including records and monitoring systems.

# And finally

It is important that as a Home Carer you recognise the need to be always aware that the level of care and assistance provided should reflect the actual needs of the person being cared for.

It is quite common for a physically and/or mentally frail person to initially need a considerable amount of intensive care, but it may be possible to reduce the level of such assistance if there is an improvement in their condition. A person with sight problems who is receiving rehabilitation training will gradually require less care, as will many people who are discharged early from hospital to recover at home.

On the other hand, someone who is relatively 'fit and able' can be provided with too much care, resulting in increased dependency rather than increased independence.

It cannot be over-emphasised – as was said at the beginning of this chapter – that all tasks should be undertaken, wherever possible, with the aim of stimulating and encouraging people to do as much as possible for themselves and increasing their independence.

The degree to which dependency is being unintentionally created can be difficult to determine, particularly if you have not worked as a Home Carer for any significant length of time.

This is an issue that should be covered in your initial training and supervision and in the monitoring and care review sessions relating to the effectiveness of the total care package for each person.

Always remember that your responsibility is not to create or reinforce dependency. You should seek to provide the level of care that is determined by the condition of the person and trigger a reassessment of need if there is a change in circumstances.

**In summary** Everyone is different and you need to adapt the care you provide to meet the individual needs of the people you care for, always ensuring that you take care to support and maintain their independence and avoid them becoming unnecessarily and inappropriately dependent.

**CHECKLIST – SUMMARY OF GOOD CARING SKILLS**

- Listening to people and what they have to say.
- Being reliable, punctual and dependable.
- Observing people and recognising when their needs change.
- Using patience, tact and persuasion.
- Avoiding confrontation.
- Recognising people's fears and frustrations.
- Putting people at ease.
- Respecting people's rights to privacy, dignity and self-respect.
- Giving essential care with gentleness, tact and confidence.
- Causing minimum discomfort.
- Recognising when to seek help from others.
- Providing care with people rather than for them.

## CASE STUDY – Mrs V

**Background**

Name: Mrs V

Age: 75

Lives alone. Supportive daughter – calls daily.

Limited mobility, due to stroke.

Problems swallowing – eats soft, chopped or liquidised food.

Medication: Various

**Care plan**

Home Carers visit three times a day, seven days a week

**Visit 1:** About 9.00 am to help get dressed, washed and help prepare breakfast.

Bath weekly, if Mrs V able.

**Visit 2:** About 12 noon to prepare and cook lunch, make a snack and leave a flask, if necessary, for afternoon tea.

**Visit 3:** About 7.30 pm to prepare supper, help get ready for bed. Secure the house.

Agency staff for domestic help weekly.

District nurses as and when necessary.

### Report 1: To the Care Manager by Home Care Manager

The home care team is finding it increasingly difficult to provide care for the above client, especially as the client and her daughter require a small nucleus of Home Carers and are unhappy with many of the staff we have previously sent.

Mrs V became a home care client on her discharge from hospital on 20 May.

Her referral asked for three visits a day:

9.00 am  1 hour to help wash/dress/breakfast.

12 noon  1 hour to prepare and cook lunch – eat soft/chopped or liquidised diet.

7.30 pm  1 hour to prepare supper and help get ready for bed.

The care plan also said that Mrs V would open the door.

Although this lady did not live in my area, I took her on short-term until more local help became available. It soon became apparent that Mrs V was unable to open the front door in the morning and that a key would have to be kept at the office to be used each day and the evening visits needed to be rescheduled for 6.00 pm. The client insists the carers arrive precisely on time. The one-hour visit was also not long enough for all the tasks to be completed to the client's satisfaction.

I had 14 Home Carers available to go into this client, and since the commencement of service, seven Home Carers are no longer able to go. Several have been requested not to visit the client for various reasons – too firm, too fat, insisting the client uses her walking frame instead of hanging on to care staff, etc. Many have just been reduced to nervous wrecks and it came to the point where their choice was either leaving home care or not going into the client again.

It is difficult to pinpoint what the problem is because if listed individually they appear minor and trivial. Mrs V elaborates problems to her daughter in order for her to remain/return. Mrs V's daughter later phones the office to report the incident and quite rightly believes her mother's account rather than ours.

We have all on several occasions met with the client and her daughter to try and resolve these issues, carefully trying to explain why we find care in this instance so difficult. However, we have failed dismally to offer the care required to the needs of Mrs V and her daughter's expectations of what we are able to offer.

Many of the problems listed below seem petty and pathetic, which is why we have never reported difficulties before. The staff also feel that singularly, each of the problems does not amount to much, but when they occur constantly during the visit the staff feel nervous, incompetent and totally inadequate.

1 Food always too hot/cold/thick/runny. Meals often have to be re-heated three times (in a microwave).
2 Client requires plates to be rinsed after washing (three times is not unknown).
3 Client waits until tasks are completed and then requests that they be redone, ie waits till all the breakfast things have been washed, rinsed, dried and put away and then says the food was too watery and has left her hungry.
4 Mrs V is very aware of the time allocated for each visit and why these constraints are necessary (ie financial as well as other client needs) but each visit usually takes longer.
5 It can take up to 40 minutes for the meal to be eaten (15 minutes when her daughter is present) and then personal care tasks follow.

**6** Blanket for legs has had to be adjusted and moved up to four times.

I was so concerned about the situation, that I asked our Training Section to arrange several sessions on anger management and this client seemed to take over the whole proceedings. The trainer was concerned about the level of stress the Home Carers were under, for whatever reason, that she suggested that individuals should keep an anger diary to complete after each visit. This has helped to a minor extent.

I am struggling to maintain some sort of continuity with the remaining seven Home Carers, but I can only send them in once a week and, therefore, problems arise when there is sickness and leave. I just need one more to drop out and I will not be able to cover the calls.

Mrs V does need continuity of care staff which I will be unable to maintain.

**This was followed by a letter to the Care Manager requesting an interim transfer of this case to agencies to enable us to schedule training and 're-grouping of staff'.**

At the case review the following was decided:

**1** Home care to provide a rota of staff two weeks in advance, so Mrs V knows which staff to expect.
**2** Home care manager requested that she visited with the care staff to observe their tasks and enable her to compile a list of procedures for all attending staff to follow.

Mrs V refused, but agreed for staff to come in pairs when new staff have to be trained, if she is given advance notice.

Mrs V to write down what she wants done, eg making Ready Brek, liquidising the meals, so all staff know the particular ways she likes things done. One copy to be kept in her home and another in home care office.

Mrs V to try a plate-warmer to keep her food hot. At present meals have to be reheated in the microwave half-way through being eaten.

During the following months there were very few weeks when Mrs V's daughter did not telephone to complain about something.

Because of the charging policy and banding, extra care hours could not be sanctioned (client refused to pay extra for her care), and staff found it almost impossible to adhere to her demands in the allotted time. Also Mrs V's condition did not improve, and staff were instructed not to leave her with any food to eat alone in case she choked.

## Conclusion

Currently there are three separate agencies coping with the care package. There are on-going problems and district nurses are also trying to resolve a complaint.

## QUESTIONS

1. How would you feel in the above situation? How long do you think you could cope in this situation?

2. What emotions and feelings do you think Mrs V is experiencing? Why do you think she is being so difficult?

3. How would you respond to Mrs V's needs? What basic skills do you think you would require?

4. Do you think this is an exceptional situation?

# KEY POINTS

- Never forget that you are working in someone else's home and treat it accordingly with care and respect. Knock or ring on the front door before entering, even if you have a key.

- You must always encourage the people you are caring for to do as much as possible for themselves to sustain their independence and enable them to remain in their own homes.

- Never impose your own personal standards; consult the person you are caring for about how they would like things to be done.

- You need to take account of health and safe working practices for your own sake, as well as that of the people you are caring for.

- Personal care tasks should always be undertaken with sensitivity and concern.

- When encouraging people to do things for themselves, allow them all the time they need. Never rush or hurry them.

- Always respect the right of the individual to choose; use persuasion to encourage attention to personal hygiene.

- Never assume that everyone is the same – we are all different.

- Always keep the person, their family and friends fully informed of what you are doing.

# 7 Health and Safety

S/NVQ Level 2: This chapter relates to the mandatory units O1, CL1, CU1 and Z1; Option Group A units Z9, Z11, Z19, W2; Option Group B units CU3, Y1.

This chapter identifies the implications for your work of the health and safety legislation and outlines what action to take in case of an accident or other emergency situation. This chapter reflects the content of *Working with Care: Health and Safety in Home Care*, a booklet produced by the Joint Advisory Group of Domiciliary Care Associations.

## Health and Safety at Work Act 1974

All employing organisations have to comply with the requirements of the Health and Safety at Work etc Act 1974. However, there are some features in relation to the provision of care to people in their own home that are beyond the scope of the Act. Also, in the case of privately provided home care, it may be the responsibility of the person receiving care to provide a safe working environment.

If you are employed directly by a local authority social services department (SSD) or a private or voluntary organisation, you are covered by the Health and Safety at Work Act. If you are registered as self-employed and paid by the person you are caring for, you are not covered by the Act. You may need to ensure that both you and the person you are caring for have adequate insurance cover in case of accidents being caused to one or other of you as the result of a mistake or negligence.

As a Home Carer you must have concern for your own health and safety as well as for those who receive your help and support, their personal family carers and their visitors. Just as in one's own home or any busy workplace, this means using commonsense, taking normal precautions and thinking ahead.

---

RELEVANT LEGISLATION

■ Health and Safety at Work etc Act 1974

■ Reporting of Injuries, Diseases and Dangerous Occurrences Regulations 1985 (RIDDOR), updated 1989

■ Control of Substances Hazardous to Health Act 1988

■ Manual Handling Regulations 1992

---

## Information on health and safety

Your organisation should have a clear policy on health and safety, which also covers manual handling. You should be given a copy of this document at the beginning of your employment and it should be regularly reviewed and updated. You should receive appropriate and necessary training as part of your induction and be familiar with the broad requirements of the relevant legislation. Home Carers need to be aware of the risks involved in providing care to people in their own homes and be able to spot potential hazards. These should immediately be referred to your line manager so that a new risk assessment may be undertaken if necessary.

Ensure that you are familiar with the health and safety policy and regulations of your employing organisation. For example, there may be specific regulations concerning the use of ladders.

## Risk assessments

The nature of home care means that you will be working in a variety of places that are not 'workplaces' in the usual sense of the word. Homes can be very dangerous places. More accidents occur in the home than elsewhere. The Royal Society for the Prevention of Accidents (RoSPA) estimated that, in 1990, there were 3.1 million accidents in the home which resulted in a recorded visit to a hospital or GP.

Before the Home Carer enters the home, a risk assessment will have been undertaken to identify the actual and potential risks to health and safety, including manual handling, involved in delivering the package of care. Your line manager should discuss and share the outcomes from this risk assessment with you before you start work in the person's home, so you both know what action and precautions you will take. If you are self-employed you should undertake your own risk assessment.

Potential hazards should always be pointed out and, if possible, discussed with the home owner in the first instance. While the principal purpose of the risk assessment is to protect you and your colleagues when providing the care, it also protects the people you are caring for. After all, anything which is a hazard to you when providing the care, is even more likely to be a hazard to the person you are caring for, when they are living all day in the home. They should be encouraged, wherever possible, to get the risks corrected – for their own personal health and safety, as well as that of others.

If the person is unable or unwilling to correct the hazard, it should immediately be reported to your line manager for appropriate action to put it right.

You must work in a safe way at all times and follow agreed safety procedures, for your own protection and that of the people you are caring for. However, the application of health and safety procedures should not infringe the rights of the people you are caring for in relation to their independence, confidentiality, privacy, dignity, choice and cultural sensitivity.

You must never use unsafe equipment. The person you are caring for has a responsibility to minimise any hazard, but cannot be required to correct it. There can therefore at times be conflict between the need to provide care services to a vulnerable person and the need to safeguard the health and safety of an employee.

The last resort is the withdrawal of care services. Naturally, agencies are extremely reluctant to do this and it should only ever happen following a full discussion with the person concerned and exploration of all possible alternatives.

**In summary** You must be fully informed of your responsibilities as a Home Carer in relation to the health and safety legislation and follow the requirements and guidelines at all times. Safe working practice in the home is vital.

# Working in a safe environment
This includes:

- Access to and exit from homes.
- The fabric of the building.
- Utilities – ie gas, electricity, water.
- Standards of cleanliness – pests and infestation.
- Pets.
- Furniture and carpets.
- Use of electrical and other equipment.
- Lifts and hoists.
- Cleaning materials.

### Access to and exit from homes

When entering a person's home, watch out for overgrown paths and slippery steps. We don't want you to have a fall before you even set foot in the house! Loose roof tiles can be a hazard to you and to others, particularly if it is windy.

Even if you have a key to let yourself in, it is good practice to knock or ring the bell first so that you don't startle your customer. It is also good practice to show your identification – at least until you know them well.

If you have a key it should be kept in a safe place when you are using it and labelled – not with your customers name and/or address but with a reference number. Your customer and your line manager should be aware of where you keep the key.

## *Fabric of the building*

Always encourage the people you care for to keep their property in reasonable condition, bearing in mind the costs involved. Your local branch of Age Concern will be able to advise you on the availability of Care and Repair schemes in your area. These schemes provide maintainence and undertake 'odd jobs' for older people at a very reasonable cost.

If the person you are caring for is in rented accommodation, you may have to ask your line manager to get in touch with the landlord to remind them of their responsibility to maintain their property.

## *Utilities – ie gas, electricity, water*

Many of the homes you visit may be old and the pipes and electrical wiring to the house may not have been renewed for a number of years. If the electrical wiring or plugs are a particular hazard, this should have been picked up when the risk assessment was undertaken.

You should be aware of the location of the taps for turning on or off any of the utilities in the homes that you visit and always follow any instructions which are supplied. If it is possible, you should advise your customers on taking out a service contract. However, the cost of this is often prohibitive.

Please discourage the people you are caring for from drying clothes close to an open fire or on top of or in front of any form of mobile heater. This can be extremely dangerous

You need to be aware of how to avoid the risk of electrical shock or fires and burns. This should be covered in your training.

You should always make use of a circuit breaker when using electrical equipment (see p 134).

## *Standards of cleanliness – pests and infestation*

As a Home Carer you will not usually be required to be part of a 'dirty homes squad' but you will sometimes work in a home that is not clean or that is in the process of being cleaned.

The question of what is clean or dirty is subjective because people have differing standards. Normally, you will be concerned to ensure that the person's home is kept reasonably clean and hygienic but this will be difficult to achieve if the person you are caring for has very poor standards.

Some very dirty homes, and people, can be caused by:

- very poor standards of hygiene and cleanliness over a long period, resulting in a dirty, smelly house;
- an 'eccentric' person whose generally poor standards are made worse by the collection and storage of rubbish such as newspapers, cans or bottles which fill the house and make cleaning impossible;
- keeping a large number of pets, usually cats and dogs, with no regard for their proper care and management.

An almost inevitable outcome of all these conditions is the infestation of the dwelling with vermin.

You should know that, in general, everyone has the right to remain in their own home, however unsanitary or hazardous the conditions. There are only two exceptions:

- People who are defined under the Mental Health Act 1983 as mentally disordered and are subject to compulsory admission to hospital.
- Under Section 47 of the National Assistance Act 1948, community physicians have powers to compulsorily remove from home people who are not mentally disordered but when it is in their own interest or to prevent injury to others. This power is very rarely used.

Most local authorities employ special teams of workers to carry out the difficult and unpleasant task of cleaning dirty premises. They are usually employed by the social services, environmental health or cleansing departments of the authority and they require special protective clothing and equipment. Some local authorities provide the services by contracting private firms.

You should:

■ Report immediately if someone's standards worsen to the point where their home is becoming dirty.

■ Seek assistance if there are signs of infestation by, for example, rats, mice, cockroaches, bedbugs, lice (animal or human).

■ Wear protective clothing if you are required to work in a dirty home or with a very dirty person (your employing agency should provide this.)

■ Seek help, advice and training on domestic hygiene and on human infestation (eg head and body lice, ringworm). You should be aware that you could become infested yourself and take appropriate precautionary measures. Your employer and your local pharmacist will advise you.

■ Be aware of the health and safety factors involved in working in dirty homes.

■ Always ensure that all your inoculations, eg for tetanus, are kept up to date.

Finally, despite the very real difficulties in working in such homes, try to maintain a sensitive approach.

## Pets

Please remember that not all pets are friendly!

Pets, particularly cats and dogs, can be a major source of pests and infestation, particularly if they have not been cared for properly and have been neglected.

It is important for you to ensure that your inoculations are up to date and that you know the correct treatment for bites, scratches and pecks. If you know you are visiting a home where there are pets who can be dangerous or playful, it may be an idea to carry a small first aid kit with you.

If there are any incidents with pets in the home, you should complete an accident report form.

If there are any signs of infestation, such as fleas and other vermin, it should be reported immediately to your line manager (see previous section).

You should be aware that pets can be a safety hazard, not only to you but also to the person you are caring for, particularly if they are unsteady on their feet. On the other hand, pets can provide comfort and company, particularly to people who live on their own.

## Furniture and carpets

Furniture and carpets, particularly if they are worn or frayed, may be significant hazards to you when working in the home. You need to know how to avoid the risk of trips and falls and never attempt to move any heavy items of furniture which may cause back injury.

Any change in circumstances or need to replace items should be reported to your line manager, bearing in mind the financial circumstances of the person you are caring for.

## Use of electrical and other equipment

Many Home Carers are now provided with residual current devices or RCDs, possibly better known as circuit breakers. If your organisation does not provide you with one, you may wish to consider investing in one yourself for your own protection.

Always use your RCD and visually check any equipment before use.

Do not overload electric points and also encourage the people you care for not to overload the points.

Always follow the manufacturer's written instructions and report any faults in the equipment to your line manager.

## Lifts and hoists

You should receive appropriate training on the use of lifts and hoists before being asked to operate this equipment, and always follow the manufacturer's instructions.

Many people needing care are reluctant to use lifts and hoists. You should explain to them that it is for their own safety as well as that of their carers. If a customer refuses to use the equipment you should report it to your line manager.

All such equipment should be regularly maintained by the manufacturer. Any failure to do so, or any defects in the equipment should be reported to your line manager and the equipment not used until it is safe to do so.

**CHECKLIST – HAZARDS IN THE HOME**

Watch out in particular for:

- Faulty electrical equipment, particularly the following:
  badly wired plugs;
  overloaded sockets;
  frayed cable;
  wrong fuse rating;
  dangerous, free-standing electric fires;
  long, trailing electrical cables.

**Note** Never take electrical equipment home with you to repair. You may be personally liable if something then goes wrong and an accident occurs.

- Faulty gas appliances (gas companies will often provide free checks for older customers).
- Be careful also of appliances using bottled gas.
- Gas taps accidentally left on.
- Mats and rugs on polished floors.
- Worn and damaged carpets.
- Dangerous and loose stair treads.
- Wet and slippery floors.
- Furniture placed in awkward positions.
- Faulty stepladders.
- Using chairs and tables in place of ladders.
- Faulty cooking utensils – eg loose handles, worn pans.
- Chipped glassware or china.
- Inadequate lighting – making it difficult to see potential hazards.
- Clothes draped over heaters to dry.

**Can you add any other items to this list?**

## Cleaning materials

You should receive training on the requirements of the Control of Substances Hazardous to Health Act in induction and be aware of the implications of the Act when handling cleaning materials.

Your employing organisation should have a policy and guidance on the use of cleaning materials which should cover, for example, the use of bleach. Please follow guidance at all times including manufacturers instructions, store chemicals in a safe place and never mix cleaning liquids or put them into unmarked or wrongly marked containers.

It is advisable to wear rubber gloves and other protective clothing whenever handling cleaning materials.

## Ensuring safe working practice

This includes:

- Basic hygiene.
- Food preparation.
- Medication.
- Moving and handling.
- Accidents and emergencies.
- Security in the home.

### Basic hygiene procedures

Always observe standard hygiene procedures to protect you and the person you are caring for against the spread of infection, and take religious and cultural needs into account.

General measures include:

- Always keep any cuts or grazes covered while they are healing. Use a waterproof adhesive dressing and replace frequently.
- Wash hands thoroughly:

- before and after contact with food;
- before and after carrying out first-aid procedures involving external bleeding and/or broken skin;
- after contact with blood or body fluids (urine, faeces, semen, vomit, sputum or tears).

■ Use disposable gloves and an apron when carrying out first-aid procedures. The gloves should be seamless, well-fitting and intact.

■ When mopping up spillage, handling heavily soiled materials or using bleach, always use household quality rubber gloves. It is a good idea to keep a different colour for different tasks, so that they can be readily identified.

■ Never share items that may become contaminated with blood (eg towels, razor blades, toothbrushes). These should be for individual use only.

## Food preparation

You should be aware of the cultural and dietary needs of the people you are caring for, and observe them at all times. Failure to do so may cause physical or psychological harm to your customers.

You need to know how to avoid infection and risk of poisoning. You also need to be aware of the effects of food allergies, for example allergy to nuts.

You should always observe the basic hygiene principals when handling food and dispose of any food which is past its 'sell by' date in a safe manner.

You will find further information on food preparation in Chapter 8, 'Eating and Nutrition'.

## Medication

Your employing organisation should have a policy on assisting with medication which you should abide by at all times.

You may be asked by the person you care for, their GP and/or district nurse to assist in helping your customers take their medication. You should only agree to do this if your line manager has been informed and you have obtained their agreement.

You will find further information on medication in Chapter 4, 'The Health of Older People'.

## Moving and handling

Thirty per cent of injuries are caused by manual lifting and handling activities. A new European Directive on manual lifting and handling came into effect in January 1993. The current legal position is that nobody should lift, move or carry a load so heavy that it is likely to cause injury.

This legislation affects your work as a Home Carer. You should receive training in lifting and handling techniques as part of your induction, but in any case you should never attempt to lift heavy loads on your own.

With the proper training, you can assist the people you are caring for and help them get in and out of a chair, bed or bath. However, you should never actually lift them yourself, even if there are two of you to do this. If lifting is required, hoists should be installed for the purpose.

Whenever lifting any object or helping the person you are caring for, you should be aware that serious injury can be caused to either or both of you if the correct procedure is not followed. In an emergency, seek help.

## Accidents and emergencies

Hopefully you will very rarely find yourself in the situation of dealing with accidents or emergencies, but it is essential that you know the correct course of action to take, if and when you do.

Accidents and emergencies come in all shapes and sizes. Some are more life-threatening, and therefore urgent, than others. In general, you are most likely to discover the accident or emergency on arrival at the person's home. The most common form of emergency is a medical emergency which may or may not have been caused by some form of physical accident. Fire, flood and burglary are other emergencies that you may encounter.

As we have already seen, very often the Home Carer will be the only person to see the person needing care on a regular, sometimes daily, basis. In earlier chapters it is emphasised that the Home Carer is often the one who is most likely to notice changes in appearance or behaviour that could indicate that the person may need help. It is not an exaggeration to say that the Home Carer can often be the 'eyes and ears' of the care agency and of health and social services departments, and can provide early warning of any problems that the person may be experiencing.

In many situations, such as an accident or burglary, it is not unknown for the person to wait for the Home Carer to arrive – someone who is familiar and trusted – before telling anyone about it.

Ideally, you should have received basic first-aid training as part of your induction training. However, realistically, this is much more likely to happen after you have been working for some length of time.

When first introduced to the person needing care (see Chapter 5), you should be informed of any pre-existing medical conditions. This should help you to understand and possibly anticipate what might happen to the person you are caring for. For example, if they suffer from diabetes (however mild) and they are found unconscious, it may be because of the diabetes. It may, however, be something else entirely, so you must always keep an open mind.

Without being intrusive and over-fussy, you should look out for the following signs when visiting each person:

- Any unexpected changes in behaviour or mood.
- Complaints of pain, giddiness or breathing difficulties.
- Untypical confusion or forgetfulness.
- Any degree of paralysis or loss of control of limbs.
- Signs of injury which may have been caused by a fall.
- Signs of non-accidental injury which might have been caused by a physical assault.
- Signs of drug or alcohol overdose.
- Burns or scalds.

The following is a checklist of the appropriate action to take if you arrive at someone's home and find them in a collapsed state or very ill.

## CHECKLIST – WHAT TO DO IN A MEDICAL EMERGENCY

- Try to stay calm, and take a few moments to plan your best course of action.
- Check that the person's airway is clear. Turn them into the recovery position if necessary.
- Never assume that the person is dead.
- Control bleeding by pressing on the bleeding point through a pad of whatever clean material is available (a towel or clean cloth, for example).
- If the person is conscious, try to get them to tell you what has happened, where it hurts, etc.
- If you think the person needs urgent attention, dial 999 and call the ambulance service without delay. Otherwise, call the person's GP.
- Do not move the person unless: to clear the airway (see above); they are in obvious potential danger (eg from fire or traffic).
- Make the person comfortable by placing a pillow under their head and covering them with a blanket. However, **do not** move the head of someone who may have injured their neck or spine.
- You should send any tablets the person is taking, and their hospital appointment card, with them to the hospital. Give these to the ambulance staff.
- Notify the GP, your line manager and any other appropriate person (eg relative or close friend), telling them of the action you have taken.

**Note** It is assumed that you have knowledge of basic first aid. If you do not, summon assistance as fast as possible and stay calm.

## CHECKLIST – INFORMATION YOU NEED TO KNOW IN AN EMERGENCY

- Basic first aid. (This should form part of your training.)
- The telephone number of key people: GP, relatives, friends, neighbours. This list should be kept in a prominent place, such as the front door or on the mantelpiece in the main living room (see Chapter 5, pp 101–103).

- Location of the nearest telephone if the person doesn't have one.
- Use of the emergency alarm, if one has been installed.
- The nearest source of help (eg neighbour, family, friend) – but don't waste time seeking this help if the situation demands a 999 call.
- In the case of fire, follow the advice of the fire service: **get out**, **stay out** and **call for help**.
- Do your best to help others get out of the property, but don't put yourself at any risk.

It is quite common now for smoke detector alarms to be fitted in homes, particularly in warden-controlled sheltered housing. These can be very sensitive and be set to go off very easily, for example by the smoke from burning toast. It would be sensible to check whether any of the homes you visit have these alarms so that you know in advance and can take any necessary action.

Slipping and falling are common accidents, particularly when helping someone to wash or bathe. To minimise the possibility of such accidents occurring, ensure that wet and dirty floors are washed and dried without delay and that suitable footwear is worn. Mats or rugs can be hazards and are easy to trip over. With the person's consent, these should be removed.

You can prevent or reduce risk of injury or infection by taking care and adopting strict standards of hygiene and cleanliness. This is particularly important when helping someone to use the toilet or when washing soiled clothing or bedding.

You should always note any points of concern and discuss these with your line manager as soon as possible. Avoid wearing jewellery, as this can cause injury.

Any accident you are involved in, whether or not it involves anyone else, must, under the requirement of the Health and Safety at Work etc Act 1974, be reported and entered into the accident report book kept by your employer. (If you are self-employed you do not need to do this, but it would be sensible for the person you are caring for to be told about the accident, if they are not already aware of it.)

These are points for general guidance. Your employing agency should have written instructions on what to do in an emergency, and telling you of this should be part of your initial training.

 **Can you think of any accident or emergency situation you have found yourself in in the past? What action did you take? Do you think it was the right action? If not, you should make sure you do know what to do next time.**

## Security in the home

You will find that some people are obsessive about security in their home, while others take a very casual approach.

As the Home Carer visiting the home, you have a responsibility to ensure that you in no way put its security at risk. If there is an agreement for you to hold a key or collect the key from a neighbour, this agreement should be in writing. Never, ever encourage someone to leave the key under the mat, on a long string inside the letter box or some other obvious place. This is an invitation to crime. Encourage them instead to obtain a 'Keysafe' home key box (see p 98).

If you think they can afford it, encourage the homeowner to have good door and window locks fitted. A peep-hole and safety chain fitted to the front door will enable them to find out the identity of callers without opening the door fully. If they are on a low income, they may be able to get assistance to improve the security of their home. The local housing department and/or crime prevention officer should be able to advise; local voluntary groups, such as Age Concern, may fit it for them.

You should also always advise the people you care for to ask for the identity card of anyone calling. Anyone – including you – on official business should have such a card.

On leaving the home, always check that the door is shut securely. If you are leaving at night, you should seek the person's permission to check that windows and all other doors to the outside are securely fastened. If you are likely to be arriving or leaving the home in the dark, you may wish to see if the person will agree to have a heat sensitive floodlight fitted – so that they can see who is at the door. It would be for their safety as well as your own. Again, the local Care and Repair scheme can assist with locks and lighting.

If someone is obsessive about security, they are likely to have a number of bolts and bars on their windows. If you arrive at the home and get no reply, try calling the person through the letter box. They may just have decided not to let you in. If they have a telephone and there is a telephone box close by, try ringing them. If there is still no reply, contact your line manager. You may need to call the police and ambulance if you think it is an emergency. On the other hand, they may have gone to visit relatives and forgot to inform the home care service!

## CASE STUDY 1

**Mrs B** is 87 years old and lives alone in a house which she owns. She has suffered a series of strokes and is confined to the ground floor. She has a colostomy which is monitored by the community nurse. The Home Carer visits mornings and evenings on seven days a week for personal care, meals and drinks.

The house is very disorganised, full of rubbish and in need of general repairs and maintenance. About 12 months ago a fire started in the living room which also affected the kitchen. The fire was thought to have been caused by the TV.

After the fire the Home Carer could not use her RCD (residual current device – see p 134) in the electric sockets. The Departmental Safety Officer inspected the premises and insisted that one socket was replaced. This was arranged by a son.

Lack of facilities and basic hygiene standards in the house cause infestation and the care manager arranges for Environmental Health to spray the premises at least three times a year.

Mrs B has a skin condition which is said to be scabies and is treated by the community nurse. She also arranges for Mrs B to be taken to a day centre occasionally for a bath.

All arrangements and incidents are recorded in the client's file.

## QUESTIONS

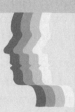

1. Identify the principal health and safety hazards you would encounter in providing care to Mrs B.

2. What particular precautions would you take?

## CASE STUDY 2

**Miss A** is 53 years old and has Down's syndrome. She has lived a sheltered life and been protected by her parents who refused all offers of help. Recently her father died and Miss A now lives with her 90-year-old mother who is also blind. There is an extended family who are very supportive.

Miss A was admitted to hospital and had cataracts removed from both eyes on the same day. The experience left her frightened and disorientated. She was unable to move. She was discharged from hospital without an assessment.

When the Home Carer arrived she found Miss A, who weighs 16 stone, in bed and soaking wet. A neighbour was present and suggested she and the Home Carer should lift Miss A out of bed. The Home Carer telephoned for assistance.

An occupational therapist and the home care manager visited immediately and a full risk assessment was completed. The recommendations were that three people were needed to move Miss A. Although a hoist may have been beneficial it was felt that Miss A would not have cooperated.

Details of the risk assessment are clearly documented and incorporated into the care plan and the client file.

## QUESTIONS

1. What are the health and safety issues incorporated in this case study? What are the risks that might be encountered?

2. What action would you take to restore Miss A's mobility and independence?

### CHECKLIST – HEALTH AND SAFETY GOOD PRACTICE

| Do | Do not |
|---|---|
| Always work in a safe manner and observe the requirements of legislation and policy and guidance of your employer. | Ever use unsafe equipment. |
| | Overload electric sockets. |
| Ensure you are covered by insurance – either your own or that of your employer. | Take someone else's equipment to your own home to repair. |
| Keep all inoculations up to date. | Mix cleaning liquids or place them in unmarked or incorrectly labelled containers. |
| Familiarise yourself with all aspects of the risk assessment. | Try to lift heavy objects unaided. |
| Report any change in circumstances affecting the health and safety of you or your customer. | |
| Use your RCD (circuit breaker). | |
| Report any faulty equipment. | |
| Wear protective clothing, including rubber gloves, whenever handling chemicals or cleaning materials. | |

## KEY POINTS

■ Always observe the correct health and safety procedures.

■ Never panic in an emergency. Assess the situation calmly before taking the appropriate action.

■ Observe any changes in the condition of the person that could indicate the onset of any medical problem or emergency.

■ Identify any major safety hazards in the home that could be a danger to you and/or the home owner. Try to persuade the home owner to get them put right.

■ Advise the home owner on ways of making the home secure.

■ Take great care when lifting. Back strain can be for life. Never attempt to lift a person yourself. Use a hoist.

■ Seek assistance if you think someone's home is becoming dirty and/or infested.

## RELEVANT ORGANISATIONAL POLICIES AND GUIDELINES

■ Health and safety – general

■ Risk assessment procedures

■ Moving and manual handling

■ Infection control

■ Cleaning of dirty and infested homes

■ Accident report procedures

■ What to do in the case of an emergency

■ Holding of keys to homes

# 8 Eating and Nutrition

S/NVQ Level 2: This chapter relates to the mandatory units O1, CL1 and Z1; Option Group A units NC12, W2; Option Group B units CU3, NC13, Y1.

This chapter looks at the importance of food to people needing care, and identifies the main components of a healthy diet. It examines some aspects of preparing meals and the range of alternative means of providing nutritious food to people who are unable to cook it for themselves. Finally, this chapter provides some guidance on helping people to eat and drink.

## Role of the Home Carer

Home Carers have an important role in promoting the health and the general wellbeing of the people they are caring for and this includes concern to ensure that they have a nutritious diet. You will be helping them with choosing, buying and preparing food, and, if necessary, helping them to eat.

Eating food is an important part of everyone's routine but meals are particularly significant for people who are housebound. Meal times should be looked forward to, and you should spend time with people while they eat.

As with all other home care activities, people being cared for should be able to choose for themselves what they wish to eat. As far as possible, they should be encouraged to prepare and cook as much of the meal as they are able themselves. Many, however, will need help.

Some people lose their appetites when they get older and may need to be tempted to eat with appetising, tasty food that they particularly like. Others may retain their appetites into very old age and have a special liking for the foods they were brought up on as children.

**In summary** You have an important role in maintaining the health of the people you care for by encouraging them to have a healthy and nutritious diet.

# The importance of a healthy diet

There is a saying that 'we are what we eat'. It is the food we eat and drink that keeps us healthy (nourishes us) and gives us energy. Too little food – or for that matter too much – can cause health problems and make us vulnerable to illness and disease.

It is advisable (although not essential) to eat a hot cooked meal every day to stay healthy, particularly in winter. A well balanced diet should contain a balance of the following foods:

- pasta or rice;
- vegetables and fruit;
- lean red meat and poultry;
- oily fish such as sardines, mackerel and tuna;
- plenty of fluids.

Foods to avoid or have in moderation include:

- any food with a high sugar content (sweets, cakes, pastry);
- saturated fat – found in butter, some cooking oils, some cheese, full cream milk;
- any fried food (grilled is healthier).

Older people, particularly those who are housebound, can be deficient in vitamin D, which is essential to keep bones healthy. This vitamin is absorbed from oily fish and breakfast cereals and from exposure to sunlight.

Think about the food you eat. Do you think that, in general, you follow a healthy diet? Could it be improved? How do you think you could best advise the people you are caring for about their diet?

If you want to find out more about healthy diets, your GP practice will be able to recommend suitable booklets or leaflets.

You should also always discuss with each individual person their personal likes, preferences and dislikes with regard to food and drink. As a general principle, everyone should be able to eat and drink whatever they choose. In time you will get to know and remember each person's likes and dislikes. But it may help to write them down first of all so that you don't forget.

You may find that some people who are housebound have little or no interest in eating because they are depressed or unhappy. It is essential to encourage them to eat by turning the meal into a social occasion and tempting the appetite with the suggestion of particular foods.

Remember the old English saying, 'a little of what you fancy does you good'. The occasional 'treat' can help sustain the older person's interest in what they are eating.

## Special diets

As part of the care plan, you should know, from the start, if anyone you are caring for has any particular dietary requirements. There may be some constraints on what the person you are caring for can eat, as a result of illness or disability.

The person you are caring for may, for medical purposes, follow a particular diet devised or recommended by their GP or a dietician. You can help by supervising the diet and encouraging the person to eat only the foods that form part of the diet.

However, no one should ever be forced or coerced into eating what they do not want. If there are difficulties, discuss them first with the person concerned. If they continue to request or eat food that is not recommended in the diet, you may need to inform the GP, nurse or dietician. But you should take this course of action only through your line manager, and you should always tell the person you are caring for what you are going to do.

Some religions have particular dietary laws and requirements that specify certain types of food – for example, Kosher and Halal. Every effort should be made to provide meals that are cooked according to the religious laws. Seek advice if necessary.

Some people you are caring for may be vegetarians or vegans (people who do not eat any animal products). Their food preferences must be respected and they should be assisted in having the food they specify. Seek help from your employing organisation if necessary.

You should also be aware of possible problems if you yourself are vegetarian or vegan and are required to cook, or to help someone eat, a meal that includes meat or animal products.

 **How do you feel about this? Would you be able to prepare the food? Remember that the person you are caring for has the same right to choose to eat meat that you have to choose not to.**

**In summary** Help people observe the requirements of any diets that they may be on for medical, religious or other reasons. Tempt people who do not feel like eating with small portions of food they particularly like.

# Buying and storing food

Allow the person you are caring for to choose what they want to eat and what you should buy. If necessary, give advice on budgeting and on the relative cost of foods. You should encourage each person to have as varied a diet as possible, within the limits of their budget.

You may need to purchase some foods that the people can prepare easily for themselves when you are not there. Remember that opening tinned food needs skill, dexterity and motivation, and this is therefore less likely to be eaten by people who do not have these abilities. An occupational therapist can advise on special tin openers that are available for people who have difficulty using standard tin openers.

Ensure that all food is stored correctly, and always in accordance with the instructions on the packaging. A person with poor vision may need help in labelling food, using either large print or braille.

If frozen food is purchased (or provided by meals on wheels), make certain that it can be stored at the correct temperature.

Regularly check the 'use by' date on all foods in the refrigerator and in the store cupboard. If there is a freezer, check the food in that as well. With the permission of the person you are caring for, place any food that is past its 'use by' date in the bin for disposal.

**In summary** Encourage people to choose the food they want to eat and buy some foods that they will be able to prepare easily themselves when you are not there. Always check that food is stored correctly and is not past its 'use by' date.

# Preparing food

Always use care when handling food. Remember to wash your hands before touching food and to always use clean containers and utensils. Follow the principles of safe hygiene practice to minimise any possibility of infection.

When preparing food, make sure it's what the person wishes to eat and cook it according to the way they want it. Present it in an attractive way and try to 'balance' it with the other meals that are likely to be taken that day. Always involve the person as much as possible in helping you prepare the food.

## Mealtimes

If your hours allow it, you should, on occasions, be present in the home when the person is eating a meal. You will provide company and stimulation, helping them to enjoy the meal all the more. It will also provide an opportunity to note discreetly exactly how much they do eat, and if they are experiencing any difficulty. For example, any difficulty in feeding themselves may indicate the onset of loss of manual dexterity or muscular control, and problems with chewing the food may indicate a need for a new set of dentures!

### People who are visually impaired

When caring for a visually impaired person, it is important to find out if they are receiving help from a rehabilitation worker in the social services department, whose job it is to teach people daily living skills within the home. If rehabilitation is being offered, you should liaise with the rehabilitation worker and see if you can assist in the programme.

If the person is not receiving help, you should find out which activities in the kitchen they feel competent to undertake and which they need help with. People with the same eye condition will vary over whether they feel confident enough to use hot saucepans, cut up vegetables or pour hot liquids. If you think the person could learn to do more themselves, you should, with their permission, seek the assistance of a rehabilitation worker.

**In summary** Always observe good hygiene practice in the preparation of food and present it in such a way that it encourages the person to want to eat.

# Alternative suppliers of meals

The meals on wheels service, day centres and luncheon clubs, family, friends and neighbours, as well as the Home Carer might provide meals when the person with care needs has difficulty in preparing food.

'Meals on wheels' may be delivered in a number of ways. The meal may be delivered already plated and 'hot', ready to eat. It may be a 'cook/chill' meal, heated up at a time to suit the service user, or it may take the form of frozen meals kept in a freezer until required.

If frozen meals are provided, make sure that the oven can be used without undue risk and that the food can be heated safely according to the instructions provided. Always check the 'use by' date on the meal to ensure it is still safe to eat. Microwaves are increasingly used to heat up ready prepared meals but many older people may need help to understand the concept of microwave cooking and be persuaded that their meal is 'properly' cooked.

The problem with most of the 'meals on wheels' is that, although they can ensure the person has a hot and nutritious meal at regular intervals, they are rarely sufficiently flexible to take into account individual food preferences.

Sometimes your role will be to supplement these sources by, for example, preparing a breakfast or supper. Where possible, and sometimes with your help, the person may be able to visit a restaurant or go for a pub lunch or have a 'take away'. It is important to try to provide 'treats' of a special meal or type of food whenever possible.

The introduction of community care and the development of flexible care packages have led to the introduction of new, flexible ways of providing meals to people in their own homes. For example, the local pub or private residential home may be contracted to deliver meals to local people, or a local ethnic restaurant may be commissioned to provide meals to a day centre or in the home for people from the same ethnic community.

**In summary** A range of meals on wheels may be available as an alternative to meals prepared by the Home Carer. Local pubs and residential homes may also deliver meals to people living in their locality.

# Alcohol

Many people enjoy drinking alcohol and this will apply to very many of the people you will be caring for.

For some, an alcoholic drink is seen either as a good appetite stimulant or as an enjoyable nightcap. If taken in excess, alcohol may cause diarrhoea, and increase the risk of falling.

There is a view that a very small intake of alcohol can be beneficial. Current health advice indicates that men should drink no more than

21 'units' of alcohol a week, and women 14. A unit is equal to half a pint of ordinary beer, or a pub measure of wine or spirits. These are the *upper* limits that are recommended.

You should remember that certain medication, especially sedatives or tranquillisers and antibiotics, may not mix with alcohol, and could cause drowsiness or, alternatively, increasing restlessness at night. You may need to remind the person you are caring for of this.

If you are concerned about the possibility of alcohol abuse (and that is not an easily defined term), it should be discussed first with your line manager before deciding on the appropriate action. It might then be mentioned to the person's GP or district nurse.

However, remember that you should always take care not to apply or impose your own personal standards and beliefs. Remember that it is always a fine balance between respecting the independence, choice, right to privacy and confidentiality of the people you are caring for and the need to refer to others such as their GP when you consider that they may be putting their health at risk.

**In summary** Watch out for signs of alcohol abuse and discourage people from taking alcohol with medication.

## Assistance with eating

Some people needing care may require varying degrees of assistance with eating. You should provide this help with tact and good humour. Remember at all times to help in such a way that it preserves the dignity of the individual person.

Where possible, meals should be provided at a time that suits each individual person, encouraging their participation in the choice of menu. The food should always be laid out so that it looks attractive and appetising to eat.

 **Think about what you like. What makes you want to eat a meal?**

Where appetite is small, as a result of little physical activity, or loss of sight, taste or smell, it is easy to be put off by the thought of a large meal. In these circumstances it is particularly important to tempt with a sample portion of the meal. After all, more can always be provided if required.

Patience and understanding are needed when helping frail people with their food. Judge whether to help with advice and encouragement, or if you need to give greater assistance. Always ask the person before cutting up food on the plate, guiding the hands or providing full assistance.

Cut up food in accordance with the wishes of the person you are assisting. If giving full assistance, always give the person exactly what they ask for. Allow plenty of time, and ensure that the person is able to indicate what they like, what they do not like and how much they want. Make sure that the food is at a suitable temperature, neither too cold nor too hot, and that you do not place the person in danger of choking by offering too large mouthfuls.

 Put yourself in the place of the person you are assisting. How do you think you would feel, not being able to feed yourself? How would you want the person helping you to respond? What would you want them to do for you?

## Aids to eating

It is important to maximise independence for people with disabilities by ensuring that appropriate eating aids are available. Where necessary, seek the help and advice of an occupational therapist or a rehabilitation worker. Care and discretion should be exercised when introducing new utensils, seeking the person's willingness to cooperate.

**In summary** Always consider the preservation of a person's dignity and respect when assisting them eat their food. Cut up the food in the way they wish and allow them the time they need to eat it and avoid rushing them. Remember to try to encourage people to feed themselves as much as possible.

# Assisting confused people

Confused older people may forget to eat and will need persuasion and encouragement to ensure that they eat regularly. People who are suffering from dementia are particularly at risk of an inadequate diet and nutrition: meals may be taken irregularly or forgotten altogether, as the sufferers have difficulty in distinguishing the time of day.

Dementia sufferers may lose weight and eat less as the illness progresses. Chewing and swallowing processes often slow down because of the difficulty in coordinating the muscles that control swallowing. Someone with a neurological condition, such as Parkinson's disease, may also have difficulty with chewing and swallowing. Allow extra time for this.

If a person totally refuses to eat, the doctor must be consulted. Encouragement should be given to take as much fluid as possible.

**In summary** You may need to use all your persuasive powers of encouragement to get a confused person to eat.

## CASE STUDY 1

**Bill** was referred to the home care service in April 1994. He was a 57-year-old man who had alcohol-related problems. He lived alone in a first floor flat in a small village.

Bill was divorced from his wife, who now lives in Australia with their two grown up children.

When Bill was first visited by the home care service he was in a dreadful state. He was drinking heavily and his personal hygiene had suffered. His flat was also very dirty and untidy.

When the home care manager first met Bill he was constantly crying and in a lot of pain with his arthritis. He was also quite objectionable and untrusting.

As the weeks went by Bill started to trust the Home Carers and actually began to enjoy their visits. Having spent quite some time talking with Bill, home care staff learned that he had had a twin brother who had died some years previously from alcohol-related problems and Bill was terrified of going the same way and dying alone.

It was suggested to Bill that he tried to stop the drinking, but he had no incentive.

Bill often spoke of his family in Australia and his big dream was to go to Australia and visit his children. Staff suggested to Bill that it needn't be a dream forever and that if he saved his money and tried to stop drinking he could probably have saved enough money to go to Australia the following summer.

Bill immediately telephoned his son in Australia and asked if he could visit him in the summer. His son was delighted at the prospect, and from that moment on Bill didn't have another drink and saved his money for his big trip. Staff were thrilled with what Bill had achieved and supported him all the way. He was very apprehensive about travelling to Australia on his own and it was arranged that he was accompanied to the airport and his son would meet him at his destination.

Bill had a wonderful time with his children that summer and was so pleased that he had fulfilled his dream.

Unfortunately, Bill started to drink very heavily on his return (a prospect that was feared, but expected) and was found dead a few days later. Unfortunately he died alone.

## QUESTIONS

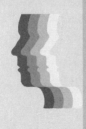

1. How would you support someone in Bill's position? What skills do you think you need?

2. How do you think Home Carers could have supported Bill on his return from Australia?

## CASE STUDY 2

**Fred**, in his early 80s, was a recent widower with diabetes who was unused to caring for himself or for the council flat in which he lived. In general, Fred was in good health and completely 'sound of mind'.

Home care was supplied three times a week and the district nurse called daily to give an injection of insulin.

One of the tasks of the Home Carers was the preparation of meals. On Fridays they would ensure that there was sufficient food for the weekend.

Over a period of time it was noticed that much of the food was left and the district nurse became concerned about Fred's weight. The situation was reported back to the manager of the home care, Fred's care manager and his GP and a case conference was held which included Fred.

Fred assured them that he was perfectly OK and was eating as much as he could. However, it was agreed that Home Carers should be present at Fred's lunchtime, five days a week. For a while all went well and after a period of some three months, the home care visits were again reduced to three days a week.

A few months later Home Carers arrived at the flat to find Fred dead. An inquest revealed that he had starved himself to death. He had gone to great lengths to hide the fact that he was not eating from both the district nurse and the Home Carers.

## QUESTIONS

1. What do you think the Home Carers could have done to encourage Fred to eat?

2. What do you think are the signs which would indicate that someone was not eating?

3. Fred was not confused. Is it his right to choose to starve himself to death if he wishes?

---

## KEY POINTS

■ You should ensure that the people you care for eat a nutritious meal at least once a day, have a varied diet and as far as possible keep to any medical diet they may be on.

■ People you are caring for should choose for themselves what they wish to eat, and, as far as possible, should be involved in its preparation.

■ Tempt people to eat by making the mealtime a social occasion, presenting the food attractively and from time to time providing food that you know they particularly like.

■ Make sure you are aware of the dietary laws and requirements of certain religions, and also of anyone who is vegetarian or vegan.

■ Always take great care when handling food and observe safe hygiene practice. Remember to wash your hands before touching the food and to use clean utensils and containers.

■ Alcohol should not be drunk if the person is on medication such as antibiotics, tranquillisers and sedatives.

■ Assist people with their food only if they really do need assistance and if they agree to you helping. Special utensils and other aids may help people with disabilities to help themselves and retain their independence.

# 9 Mobility and Disability

**S/NVQ Level 2: This chapter relates to the mandatory units O1, CL1, OU1 and Z1; Option Group A units Z6, Z7, Z9, Z11, Z19, W2; Option Group B units Y1, Z5.**

Mobility means simply the action of getting from one place to another.

Keeping mobile and active is very important. Different people require differing degrees of help to remain mobile and their needs may vary over time. Mobility can easily decrease and dependence increase if people are left to sit around their homes for long periods.

As a Home Carer you have a responsibility to do everything you can to maintain and support the people you are caring for and to ensure that they retain the maximum amount of independence possible in their lives. Mobility is a very important factor in maintaining independence.

## Physical difficulties experienced by older people

Older people frequently experience certain physical difficulties which may become disabilities and lead to a loss of mobility. These include difficulty with:

- walking, which can lead to the need for walking aids and possibly, eventually, a wheelchair;
- failing sight, causing lack of confidence in moving inside and outside the home;

- using hands, especially for grasping, opening things, using switches, dressing, going to the toilet;
- getting in or out of bed or the bath;
- climbing stairs and negotiating furniture;
- walking outside of the house, leading to a lack of confidence in crossing roads and busy junctions.

**In summary** Be alert to signs of disability which may lead to a decrease in mobility.

## The importance of mobility

The quality of life for some older people can worsen because they become housebound and isolated. This can happen over a long period, beginning with a disabling illness or accident or as the result of the death of a partner.

Older people, just like anyone else, can become depressed. However, it is easier for the cycle of depression to become self-reinforcing for older people. They can't be bothered to go out so they begin to lose their social skills and their mobility. The less they get out to shops, to see friends, to go to bingo or to church or the theatre, the less they become able to.

With appropriate professional advice you can help to halt this process and, if needed, with appropriate aids, can begin to restore mobility and confidence. People with failing sight can be referred to a rehabilitation worker for an independent assessment.

A positive approach to the provision of care can help to restore interest and purpose to the person's life. A balance must be struck between the real limitations of each individual and their actual potential abilities. This balance should be identified by all the people involved in decisions relating to the provision of care services – including the person needing care and any personal carers they may have, such as family and friends.

If care and help are being provided through the local authority social services department or the local community health trust, each person being cared for should have a personal care plan. Decisions that are reached concerning the most effective means of maintaining the independence and mobility of the older person should be included in the care plan.

Before starting to provide care, managers need to obtain detailed information about the capability of each person - this should form part of the care plan. This information must be shared and discussed with you, the person directly providing the care. Only then will you have sufficient knowledge of the person's needs to give the appropriate level of care and support. Ideally, a copy of the care plan should be left in the home for carers to refer to. However, it is known that some social services departments are reluctant to share the full contents of the care plan with agencies external to the local authority who are contracted to provide the care.

It is, however, a mistake to give too much help. It must be remembered that some instructions given as part of a care plan can seem harsh and uncaring, but they are vital to encourage independence. Dependency can be increased if help is always given to get out of a chair or to walk. In such cases, some individuals will quickly lose the will to move around independently.

Wherever possible, you should help and encourage each person to do as much as they can for themselves. This is not always easy. They may have already become dependent and it is not unknown for even relatively fit older people to expect to be 'looked after' in their later years. It is, however, better for their general state of health and personal confidence if you encourage them to help with making the bed, dusting and food preparation rather than to do these tasks for them.

**In summary** Loss of mobility increases dependence. You therefore need to encourage the person to do as much as possible for themselves and involve them, whenever possible, in the tasks you are undertaking.

**CHECKLIST – EXAMPLES OF WAYS OF ENCOURAGING MOBILITY**

- It is generally better to encourage a person to rise from a chair unassisted if they can.
- It may be more helpful to walk alongside a person without physically supporting them if they can manage.
- Allow people with visual loss to say how they wish to be guided.
- Wheelchairs must not be used merely to save time.
- Try to provide moral rather than physical support.
- Be aware when to be firm or gentle, or to negotiate.
- Show sympathy and praise effort. (Constant chivvying can be irritating and counter-productive.)
- Involve the person in undertaking tasks around the home; don't let them sit in a chair and watch you do it all.
- Put on some music and encourage them to move in time to it.
- Ensure that walking frames, when used, are always within reach, and are correctly adjusted to suit the height of the individual.
- An armchair suited to an individual's needs can make all the difference in enabling them to sit down and get up unaided.
- Wheelchairs and other equipment should be regularly inspected and maintained.[11]
- Be aware of safe practices when using walking aids or wheelchairs, and pass this information on to users, wherever possible.

# The importance of exercise

Exercise is important at any age, and most of us don't get enough of it. A certain amount of exercise, adapted to meet the particular needs of each person you are caring for, will improve strength, suppleness and stamina.

Try putting the radio or other music on and encouraging the person to move and 'dance' to the music. Keep-fit and music-and-movement exercises are good ways of encouraging mobility. You may

---

11 If issued by the Disablement Services Authority, inspection should be carried out by the designated approved repairer. This information should have been given to the person at the time the wheelchair was issued.

find that these activities take place in a local day centre or residential home, and the person may be able to join in – although transport may have to be arranged.

Swimming is very good exercise at any age, but in particular for anyone who is overweight or has back problems or disabilities, as the water supports the body.

**In summary** Use music to encourage even the most gentle exercise.

# Care of feet

The single most important aid to mobility are the feet. Good foot care is therefore essential for maintaining mobility and general functioning and therefore independence. Many problems with the feet can be prevented; whenever possible you should encourage the people you are caring for to wear properly fitting shoes that provide support, rather than slippers, as normal footwear.

If anyone you are caring for has any problems with their feet, including corns, ingrowing toenails, hard skin or is experiencing pains in their feet when walking, encourage them to see a chiropodist. Many are willing to make home visits and if you tell the GP what the problem is, they will generally pass on the referral to the NHS chiropodist.

You may need to wash a person's feet if they are unable to do so themselves. Take great care to dry between the toes as this can be a source of infection. Never cut toenails or attempt to treat corns. These must be done by a chiropodist because an accidental cut to the skin can cause infection, ulceration and even gangrene. People with diabetes or circulatory problems are particularly at risk. The chiropodist can also advise on the proper footwear.

**In summary** Taking care of the feet is a major aid to sustaining mobility and therefore independence.

# Equipment that assists mobility

Local authorities (usually through their social services departments) and health authorities can provide a range of equipment which will help people to cope with different kinds of disabilities. The equipment and adaptations that are generally available include:

- **Walking aids** such as sticks, pulpit (Zimmer) frames, crutches and wheelchairs. Assessment of need, help and advice on their use are available from physiotherapists, occupational therapists and/or aids assistants. As a general rule, the person should be encouraged to manage with the most simple aid that meets their needs, to avoid the danger of increasing dependency. For example, use one walking stick rather than two or use two walking sticks rather than a Zimmer.
- **Symbol canes or long canes** for people with poor sight who have received mobility training.
- A wide range of **devices that help in reaching and grasping objects,** in opening bottles and jars, in cooking and preparing food and drinks, and in dressing.
- Various types of **lifts** to enable people to go up and down stairs.
- General **adaptations to the person's home** to make it more easily accessible to them (eg ramps, downstairs toilet/bathroom, adapted kitchen).
- **Aids and equipment to assist toileting and bathing,** including hoists and sometimes the installation of a shower.
- **Aids for people with poor vision.** Also check on lighting and encourage the use of colour contrast (eg a red jug on a white surface is easier to see than a white jug on a white surface).
- **Incontinence accessories** and supplies (see also Chapter 10).

You need to know the range of aids that are available, their function and where they can be obtained. Consult your line manager and/or occupational therapist if you think any special equipment may assist the person you are caring for.

The Disabled Living Foundation (address in Appendix 8) provides comprehensive information on all the equipment and aids that are available to assist people with daily living. The Royal National Institute for the Blind (address in Appendix 8) has information on aids for people with poor vision.

Some places in the country have special community transport

schemes to take people with disabilities and their carers to the shops. Many large shopping centres operate 'Shopmobility' schemes which provide wheelchairs to assist people who are not very mobile. You should be aware of whether any of these schemes operate in your area and be able to advise the people you are caring for accordingly. Your local branch of Age Concern will be able to provide you with information.

**In summary** There are a range of aids and adaptations which assist mobility. You need to be generally aware of the ways in which they could assist the people you care for, including the existence of any local community transport and shopmobility schemes.

## Care of pressure areas

People who lack mobility – for whatever reason – and spend long periods sitting in chairs or lying in bed are prone to develop pressure sores. These occur where any bony point presses against an underlying surface. People who are very thin or obese, suffering from incontinence or poor circulation and are unable to move themselves easily are particularly likely to develop pressure sores.

You will need to understand the principles of care of pressure areas and the prevention of sores. However, Home Carers should carry out care of pressure areas only under the supervision of a district or community nurse and only after having the appropriate training.

Prevention of pressure sores is helped by:

- a good diet;
- ensuring absolute cleanliness of the skin (especially if the person is incontinent – see also Chapter 10);
- moving the person's position every 2–3 hours to promote circulation;
- keeping bedding and other covers smooth and free from crumbs;
- avoiding friction in lifting.

If soreness occurs, the GP may prescribe cream for application to the infected area.

Pressure-relieving aids such as sheepskins, anti-pressure pads, urine-absorbing sheets and 'ripple pads' and mattresses can be helpful.

**In summary** If you are caring for people who are immobile, watch out for signs of pressure sores and report them to your line manager and/or the district nurse.

## CASE STUDY 1

**Mr and Mrs L** had lived together for many years and were in their late 60s. Mr L had taken early retirement at the age of 52 to look after his wife who was becoming increasingly disabled owing to arthritis. As Mrs L's condition continued to worsen, she had severe walking difficulties, and her hands and knuckles became swollen and very painful. Her husband 'did everything for her', and she had become dependent, losing all motivation to help herself. The couple had not sought, nor had they received, any assistance from social services. They had no close family, and Mr L had for years prided himself on his ability to care for his wife without outside help.

Mr L died of a heart attack at the age of 69. Suddenly, Mrs L was deprived of the love and support of a long-term carer; she had little ability or motivation to help herself. She was referred by neighbours to the GP and social services.

There was a swift assessment of Mrs L's needs and, with her agreement, she was admitted to hospital for an in-depth review of her condition, medication and level of functioning. Upon her discharge, there was an assessment by all agencies involved, in her own home, of her ability to cope. Various aids were provided, and Mrs L received occupational and physiotherapy support and treatment aimed at developing her independence. Throughout the whole process, Mrs L had been allocated a Home Carer to provide help and support as she tried to establish herself in her own home. After a period of three months, Mrs L became able to care for herself with the services of a Home Carer visiting three times a week and with some other domiciliary services.

## QUESTIONS

1 What individual skills do you think the Home Carer used in caring for Mrs L?

2 Should somebody be aware of cases where a disabled older person is cared for by a single carer, so that problems may be anticipated?

3 If Mrs L had not improved sufficiently to be able to care for herself at least partially, what do you think would have been the outcome?

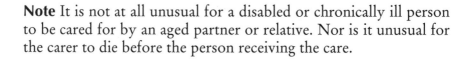

**Note** It is not at all unusual for a disabled or chronically ill person to be cared for by an aged partner or relative. Nor is it unusual for the carer to die before the person receiving the care.

## CASE STUDY 2

**Mrs J**, at 89 years old, was able to manage by herself without support until she had a stroke. She was admitted to hospital but was making very slow progress. There was considerable pressure on the hospital beds at the time and it was agreed that Mrs J would be discharged. She would attend the day hospital for physiotherapy when a place could be arranged.

Once home, Mrs J was confined to the first floor of her house. Having got upstairs with assistance, she was unable to get down again and she could not access the bathroom. She quickly became very distressed and the Home Carers who visited five times daily were very concerned.

The Home Carers consulted their line manager who arranged a visit from the community occupational therapist (OT). The OT arranged to provide various daily living aids and worked out a programme of rehabilitation in which the Home Carers would participate.

Mrs J was very pleased and worked very hard to regain her mobility, with the support of the Home Carers. Within three weeks she could manage the stairs again. A further three weeks of constant practice followed and Mrs J was able to attend to all of her own personal care needs and prepare her own meals.

Mrs J continues to need some support with housework and shopping; however, she is looking forward to taking over her domestic tasks in the near future although she will probably need longer-term support for shopping.

## QUESTIONS

1. What arrangements should have been made on Mrs J's discharge from hospital?

2. As Mrs J's Home Carer, what would you do to assist her regain her mobility?

3. What may be Mrs J's needs in the longer term?

## KEY POINTS

- Mobility is a key factor in maintaining independence.
- Involve the person in doing tasks around the home, in order to increase their mobility.
- Encourage the person to do simple keep-fit exercises.
- Make sure that care is taken of the feet and encourage the wearing of properly fitting shoes that provide support.
- Encourage the use of simple aids to assist mobility. Avoid the use of aids that are not necessary, as they will only increase dependence.

# *10* Maintaining Continence

**S/NVQ Level 2:** This chapter relates to the mandatory units O1, CL1 and Z1; Option Group A units Z7, Z9, Z11, Z19, W2; Option Group B units CU3, Z8.

To many people, the maintenance of continence is important to their self-respect and self-image. It is therefore very important to be able to help people to find ways to maintain continence, as this in turn affects the rest of their wellbeing and general approach to life.

Incontinence should never be accepted as just 'part of getting old'.

Incontinence may occur at any age. It is not inevitable in old age but it does occur in both men and women and it can be a cause of great embarrassment and loss of self-esteem and self-confidence. Yet it can frequently be easily cured or at least improved by very simple measures. Whatever can be done to minimise its effect is always of great benefit to sufferers and their personal carers.

## The onset of incontinence

Home Carers may be the first to notice the onset of incontinence because of their regular contact with the people they are caring for.

Incontinence can be treated and in most cases, with proper management, the condition can be greatly improved or even cured. Maintaining continence should always be the main aim.

The sufferer may be incontinent of urine or faeces or both. Incontinence may be temporary – for example, due to infection or to emotional disturbances such as bereavement. It may, however, indicate the onset of deterioration of intellectual functioning (dementia).

Incontinence should always be referred to the GP, who may involve a specialist incontinence adviser – generally a district nurse.

Tact and discretion should be used to discuss the issue of incontinence with sufferers. They should be encouraged to seek medical help themselves, if at all possible.

People are very frequently ashamed of being incontinent. It is not unknown for people to go to considerable and sometimes bizarre lengths to hide the evidence of their incontinence, which may include hiding soiled clothing. This is often an indication that the person is aware that they are not managing to cope with this aspect of their life. Try to show understanding of the problem and acceptance of the reasons for it. This will encourage the sufferer to do something about it.

If the sufferer takes no action themselves, even with encouragement, and does not contact their GP or district nurse, you should report the situation to your line manager – but make certain that your client knows this is what you are going to do.

Even when it is not possible to make significant improvements in the condition, the tactful and sympathetic care that you and others provide can do a great deal to reduce the physical and emotional discomfort caused by the condition.

**In summary** Use tact and discretion when raising the subject of incontinence with the people you are caring for – be sympathetic and understanding.

# Causes of incontinence

There is often no single cause of incontinence. It generally arises from a combination of both physical and environmental factors, most of which are not irreversible.

**Physical** factors include:

- urinary tract infections;
- diabetes;
- after-effects of a stroke;
- enlarged prostate gland (in men);

- some neurological conditions or infections can result in a loss of control;
- severe constipation;
- stress incontinence (a leakage of urine caused by a sneeze or a cough);
- drugs, such as:
  - sedatives and tranquillisers which diminish the sensation of needing to pass urine, and get to the lavatory in time;
  - diuretics (water tablets), given to people for a number of conditions (including heart failure) to increase the ability of the body to rid itself of fluids;
  - alcohol is also a diuretic, and drinking a large quantity of beer, etc, can cause a loss of control.

**Psychological** factors include:

- anxiety;
- changes in lifestyle;
- worry over not being able to reach the lavatory in time and 'having an accident';
- loss of self-esteem and self-confidence;
- imagined or actual rejection by relative;
- stress or bereavement;
- a form of anger against the circumstances of life.

**Environmental** factors include:

- lack of easy access to a lavatory (eg lavatory upstairs);
- inadequate lighting and heating in the lavatory;
- lack of handrails and aids to ensure that the lavatory seat is at the right level;
- concern about arrangements during the night and reluctance to use a commode;
- inability to get out of bed at night and use the commode;
- concern about any lack of privacy, particularly when help has to be given in toileting arrangements;
- difficulties in removing clothing in time.

**In summary** There are many physical, medical (drug-related), psychological and environmental factors which can contribute to the cause of incontinence.

**CHECKLIST – ACTION YOU CAN TAKE TO IMPROVE CONTINENCE**

- Encourage attention to diet and adequate intake of food and drink.
- Do not restrict intake of liquids during the day, other than alcohol, as this can lead to dehydration.
- Avoid taking too many drinks in the evening, before going to bed.
- Try to ensure that any drugs prescribed are taken as indicated.
- Encourage regular visits to the lavatory and, in particular, at bed times (part of a continence programme).
- Try to ensure that lavatory facilities are within easy reach.
- Encourage independence in the use of the lavatory.
- Afford as much privacy as possible when helping the sufferer to the lavatory.
- Arrange for the provision of mobility aids if it is difficult to reach the toilet in time.
- Avoid too much preoccupation with the condition and paying too much unnecessary attention to it.
- Avoid any form of conflict over the condition – that will only make the situation worse.
- Keep the sufferer clean and dry.
- Work with others involved – for example, the GP, nurse, continence adviser – to maintain an agreed continence programme (as it is called).
- Advise health staff if there are any changes in the condition.

Generally:

- Always help the sufferer in a way that will maintain their privacy and dignity at all times.
- Do not discuss the person's incontinence with a third person present unless they are there to give medical advice.
- **Never** blame the sufferer when accidents occur nor make them feel embarrassed or ashamed in any way when you are changing pads or washing them.
- **Never** let the sufferer feel that you find these activities distasteful. Be aware of the feelings that may be experienced owing to incontinence – fear of reprimand, shame, embarrassment, loss of self-control and loss of dignity. Acknowledge them as sensitively as possible. To ignore them could increase the problem.

■ Try to reassure the sufferer that incontinence does not damage the respect that they deserve as an individual.

**In summary** There are a number of ways in which you can help people maintain their continence – you need to be familiar with them.

# Sources of help

You should never feel isolated and unsupported in any aspect of the care you provide, and this applies to the challenging area of maintaining continence and improving incontinence. Help and support should be available from the following sources/people:

■ Health service staff, particularly district nurses, occupational therapists and continence advisers, who are employed by many health authorities.
■ On a practical level, supplies of various aids, such as special clothing, pads, pants, waterproof sheets, commodes, raised lavatory seats, drawsheets and mattresses, should be available from the health service or, in some cases, from the local authority social services department.
■ Handrails may need to be fitted, or special toilet seats installed.
■ Clothing that can be unfastened quickly and easily may help.
■ Exercises can strengthen bladder control. Information on these may be obtained from the district nurse and/or physiotherapist who should meet the sufferer and assess their need.
■ Where sufferers have to be fitted with a catheter, help and advice on management will come from health service staff.
■ Your own agency may have guidelines on maintaining continence, which should be easily available. Check with your line manager.
■ Training should be available for home care staff working with people suffering with incontinence.

**In summary** You need to be familiar with the sources of help available to maintain continence. You should also receive training.

# CASE STUDY 1

**Mr M,** in his mid-70s, lived with his daughter in a house with an upstairs toilet. For some years he had experienced increasing difficulty in passing urine. He got to the point where he had to go very frequently during both day and night; he rarely thought that he had emptied his bladder; urine flow was retarded and slow. He got little warning before needing to go to the toilet. Sometimes he began to pass urine before he reached the toilet or his underwear became stained because he 'dribbled' after emptying his bladder.

He became miserable and ashamed of this; he worried that his daughter might find out about what he considered to be his urinary incontinence. He was a very private man who did not like the idea of discussing his problem with anyone, least of all with his daughter. She was aware of his difficulties but did not feel comfortable about mentioning it to him.

His daughter had a job that required occasional travel abroad. On these occasions a Home Carer was provided to help Mr M. The Home Carer became so concerned about Mr M's condition that she asked Mr M whether he had sought help. For the first time, Mr M was able to unburden himself about what he considered to be a shameful situation. The Home Carer persuaded Mr M to see his GP; he was referred to hospital and was treated for the effects of an enlarged prostate gland. After convalescence, his 'problem' was very much improved.

## QUESTIONS

1. What interpersonal skills do you think the Home Carer used?

2. What does the case study tell you about communication in the M family?

3. Why do you think that for some people a problem like this is 'shameful', while other people would think little of it and see a GP as soon as the condition became troublesome?

4. If the problem had not been so easily resolved, how do you think Mr M could have been helped?

## CASE STUDY 2

**John** has cerebral palsy and has lived in hospital for most of his 28 years. His circumstances were brought to the attention of a physiotherapist who shared John's view that he could live independently in the community. This was contrary to the view of other health and social care professionals who had been caring for John in the institution for many years.

After a long uphill struggle, John eventually moved into an adapted bungalow in a sheltered housing scheme with an intensive package of care.

John's case was an enormous success and a great achievement for all involved, particularly John himself. In his new-found freedom John exerted his choice over many things, including his choice of food. He would not be advised. As a result he put on so much weight that the Home Carers were having difficulty getting him in and out of his wheelchair. His poor diet affected his bowel movement and he was continually calling the warden and mobile wardens to assist him after his many 'accidents'. John's independence was becoming seriously threatened.

A planning meeting was arranged and John attended, as did the Home Carers. John's problems were honestly discussed. John asked the Home Carers to plan and control his diet and agreed to co-operate.

John lost weight and his bodily functions were restored to a regular routine which co-incided with the visits of the Home Carers. John continues to live happily in his own home.

## QUESTIONS

1. What do you think would be the particular care needs that John would have?

2. How would you approach the issue of maintaining continence?

## KEY POINTS

- Incontinence can often be cured or at least improved. It should never be accepted as an inevitable part of growing old.
- People are frequently embarrassed and ashamed about being incontinent. You should show tact and sympathy, and understanding and acceptance of the reasons for it.
- Take appropriate action to minimise the effect of incontinence.
- Seek assistance from the incontinence adviser and other health service professionals.

# *11* Financial Matters

**S/NVQ Level 2: This chapter relates to the mandatory units O1, CL1 and Z1; Option Group A unit W2; Option Group B unit Y1.**

This chapter considers issues relating to the personal finances of people receiving care, including charging for the service. It explores the level of involvement that Home Carers should have with the personal finances of those they are caring for and what happens if people are unable to look after their own finances themselves.

## Personal finance

People receiving care should always be encouraged to take full responsibility for handling their own financial affairs and have the right to choose and control how their money is spent. Some people, however, although capable of managing their own affairs, receive assistance from relatives, friends or solicitors.

Someone who is physically frail and housebound may choose to:

1. Draw up a mandate, authorising another person to use their bank or building society account to carry out essential transactions.
2. Authorise an agent to act on their behalf – for example, with the agreement of their employing organisation, authorising a Home Carer to collect their pension by signing the appropriate slip in the pension book.
   **Note** It is always possible nowadays, and generally preferable, to have the pension paid directly into an account in a bank or building

society – there is no need any longer to have to spend time collecting it in person from the Post Office

3. Appoint another person, generally a relative or a solicitor, to act on their behalf through a 'Power of Attorney' (see p 182).

4. Authorise another person, generally a relative, to act as the 'Appointee' on their behalf, to make claims and receive benefits on behalf of the claimant from the local Benefits Agency (Social Security office).

Inevitably you will find that you almost always have to deal with money belonging to the person you are caring for, even if it is only the fairly basic level of shopping, reading bills for someone who has poor vision, paying bills or collecting pensions. It is clearly an area where difficulties can arise and you should be aware of the need to be _extremely careful._

Responsible agencies employing Home Carers should have their own guidance on money matters. If you belong to a trade union, this may also be a source of specific advice. Age Concern Books have published a helpful reference book, _Managing Other People's Money_, by Penny Letts (see p 245). The following general guidelines are intended to warn you about the potential pitfalls, bearing in mind that you might be dealing with the finances of people who may be forgetful, vulnerable or confused.

## Level of involvement

Shopping, paying bills and collecting pensions are of considerable help to many people. These tasks may be part of your work, where it has been assessed as a care need and is part of the care plan.

Any further involvement beyond this level (for example using banking services, making withdrawals from Post Office Savings or building society accounts) should be resisted. Any request that you undertake more than basic financial transactions on behalf of the person you are caring for should be discussed with your line manager.

## Providing financial advice

You may find that the people you are caring for need advice and assistance in budgeting. Advice may be offered on how to allocate weekly spending to cover essential items such as food, fuel bills, rent, etc, and ways explored of spreading the payment of bills by (for example) the purchase of TV, telephone or electricity stamps or other similar budget payment schemes. The Post Office and the Citizens Advice Bureau will have leaflets on budget payment schemes. Gas and electricity companies offer a range of payment methods; some of these (such as prepayment meters) are more expensive than either quarterly bills or monthly direct debit payments from a bank account – there is often a reduction for payment by direct debit.

You may need to seek advice from the Department of Social Security/Benefits Agency, Citizens Advice Bureau or Age Concern if you think someone is not claiming all the benefits to which they are entitled, for example Attendance Allowance.

## Shopping

When purchasing items on someone else's behalf, each item should be discussed, including its general availability, where to buy it and the likely cost. This is particularly important if the person has been housebound for some time and has no recent experience of shopping for the items concerned. You should make alternative suggestions, if appropriate, so that the person can make an informed choice on how to spend their money.

Ensure that the person knows exactly how much of their money you are taking to do their shopping – ensure that the amount is written down and agreed by both parties. Always keep the other person's money entirely separate from your own.

When actually doing the shopping, make certain a written record is kept of all transactions. If shopping in a modern supermarket, the receipt provides a detailed breakdown of all purchases. If shopping on a regular basis, it is a good idea to keep a notebook in the home, especially for the purpose of keeping a written record.

When returning with the shopping, go through the cost of each purchase in turn with the person you have bought it for. Account for all money spent and count out the change into the person's hand. Ensure they are comfortable with the amount you have spent and the change they have received.

Dealing with money can be a particularly sensitive area when the person has visual difficulties. You might ask them to take the money out of their purse themselves and hand it to you. Similarly when giving back change, it is advisable to count it back into the person's hand so that they know exactly what change you have given them. The Royal National Institute for the Blind provides aids to assist people with poor sight to identify their money.

**In summary** Take great care when handling money belonging to someone else. Never mix it up with your own money and account for all expenditure in writing. Keep records of expenditure. Be aware of sources of information to assist with budgeting.

# Valuable possessions

Everyone has the right to dispose of their own personal valuables, such as jewellery, as they wish. Some may have made arrangements with banks for safe-keeping. Others may not be aware of the value of their possessions and leave them around the home for everyone to see.

If you are worried about the security of valuable items or of large sums of money kept in the house, you should discuss it first with the person concerned – including the possible physical danger to themselves as a result of theft and burglary. This should be done calmly and factually, without causing any alarm but alerting them to the dangers they are placing themselves in.

If you continue to be worried, the situation should be discussed with your line manager and, with the agreement of the person concerned, with their relatives.

## *Accepting gifts*

Many of the people you are caring for will be very grateful for your help, support and care, and will wish to show their gratitude. You must be very, very careful about accepting gifts. You will need to use your discretion in deciding whether or not to accept gifts. To refuse could give offence, but to accept a too extravagant or expensive gift could be interpreted as improper conduct. Your employing organisation may have a specific policy relating to the acceptance of gifts – find out if they have.

In general, acceptance of a small, modest gift on birthdays or at Christmas should not be misconstrued. If you are in doubt, discuss it with your line manager. As a rough 'rule of thumb' some organisations allow gifts up to about £5 in value, but no more.

If the person you are caring for suggests mentioning you in their Will, you should take positive steps to discourage them and inform your line manager. To seek a bequest in their Will would be quite improper.

**In summary** Alert people you care for to the dangers of leaving valuable possessions lying around the home. Only accept small gifts from the people you care for, £5 or less in value. Never seek to be mentioned in their Will.

# Inability to manage personal finances

Some people may be or become unable to manage their own financial affairs because of confusion or other mental disability. In these cases, arrangements will have to be made for others to act on their behalf. The person taking responsibility for the financial affairs may be a relative, friend or solicitor. However, if there is no-one able or willing to undertake the duties of an Attorney (see p 179) or a Receiver (whichever is appropriate in the circumstances) you will need to contact the local authority to enquire if a member of their staff undertakes these roles for people in this position. (See following section on 'Enduring Power of Attorney'.)

It is a major decision to remove a person's right to manage and handle their own finances and must never be taken lightly. Every effort must be made to safeguard their best interest.

You may consider that someone you are caring for is reaching the stage of confusion where they are unable to handle their finances. Report this to their relatives and to your line manager, who will, if necessary, arrange for an assessment (including a psychiatric assessment) to be made by the appropriate people.

## *Enduring Power of Attorney*

Any arrangements the person had previously made for managing their affairs, such as an ordinary Power of Attorney (see p 179), will cease to be valid, unless an Enduring Power of Attorney (EPA) order has been made.

An EPA should be created while the person (the 'donor') is still capable of understanding the nature and effect of creating such a document when it is explained to them. For example, the 'donor' should know that the attorney will be able to assume complete authority over their *financial* affairs and will be able to continue to deal with these matters even when the donor is no longer able to supervise the attorney's actions. If the donor is able to understand the role of an EPA, the fact that the donor may, at the same time, be 'incapable by reason of mental disorder of managing and administering their property and affairs' does not affect the validity of the EPA. The EPA should be registered with the Court of Protection as soon as it has been signed by the donor and the attorneys.

The EPA can come into effect immediately it has been signed by the donor and attorney, or after it has been registered with the Court of Protection, depending upon the wording of the EPA. In either case, as soon as the attorney has reason to believe that the person is or is becoming mentally disordered, the attorney must apply to the Court of Protection to have the EPA registered. It is not necessary to have the mental incapacity formally diagnosed.

The person who holds the EPA has to take out insurance to protect the person's finances – the cost met by the 'donor'.

With the policy of care in the community there are likely to be an increasing number of cases where it is possible to provide support to enable people to live at home, but who cannot manage their own personal finances.

### Court of Protection

If the person has assets, it will be necessary to apply to the Court of Protection. If the person's assets are small, the Court of Protection may issue a Short Procedure Order enabling someone to deal with these. However, if the assets are substantial, the Court has the power to appoint a Receiver to control and manage the person's finances and property on their behalf. It is likely that a member of the person's family would be appointed as the Receiver.

As the Home Carer you will be in a position to provide valuable information about the person you are caring for and about their physical and mental condition. However, if you are concerned, it should be discussed with your line manager, who can ensure that appropriate steps are taken. You should not take direct action yourself in these circumstances.

If there is no relative or friend willing and able to act as Receiver, the court will appoint a solicitor. Application proceedings are slow but may be speeded up in certain circumstances.

Further information on management of financial affairs is provided in Age Concern Factsheet 22 *Legal arrangements for managing financial affairs* (details on p 239).

**In summary** An Enduring Power of Attorney order may be made to assume responsibility for a person's financial affairs should they subsequently become confused and unable to continue to be responsible themselves. A Court of Protection will safeguard a person's assets and possessions.

# Charging for the service

Most social services departments make some charge for the provision of home care. This may be:

1. A flat rate charge to all, irrespective of how many hours of service are actually provided.
2. A tiered charge dependent upon the number of hours of service provided.
3. A tiered charge dependent upon the income of the person needing care and their ability to pay.

Many local authorities do not charge people for the service if they are on Income Support, but they do charge if the person is in receipt of Attendance Allowance.

## Financial assessment

In general it will be the care manager who will undertake the financial assessment as part of the care plan and package. It will be their responsibility to ensure that the person fully understands what they should pay and signs the necessary forms, before you commence providing the care service.

Nevertheless, whether you are employed by the social services department, or your organisation is contracted to provide services on behalf of the SSD, or you are employed and paid privately for the care you provide, you should be aware of the basis upon which the charges are made to the person you are caring for.

People receiving care are entitled to a full explanation of the mechanism for charging for the service. They also have the right to choose whether or not to have the service, on the basis of cost.

If you work for a private agency which provides home care services on behalf of the local authority social services department, you may be expected to collect the financial contribution on a regular basis from the people you are caring for and pass it on to your agency as part of the contract with the local authority. Although by no means an ideal method of collection, or one that would be recommended, it is known to occur. If you are expected to collect the money, ensure that you have a record of receipt signed by both parties, and that you are able to keep it somewhere safe. Always pass the money over to the agency on the day you receive it.

# Welfare rights

Many people may be entitled to benefits such as Income Support or Housing or Attendance Allowance. People aged under 65 may be eligible for a Disabled Living Allowance. Because you are frequently the one person who is in most regular contact with the person needing care, you will often be asked for advice and information on a wide range of subjects, including benefits.

You should check with the person that they are aware of all the possible entitlements. This may have been undertaken originally by the care manager when assessing need, but benefits and entitlement change. You can help by obtaining relevant information leaflets on their behalf and, if appropriate, making contact with welfare rights advisers, the Department of Social Security/Benefits Agency and other agencies giving specialist advice.

You should be aware that Attendance Allowance and Disability Living Allowance are given to people so that they can purchase the additional care they need – this may include home care. Some of the people you care for may be asked by the local authority to contribute part, or even all, of their Attendance Allowance to pay for the range of care services they receive in their own home. If this has not happened before, it may be initially resented. You need to be aware that this is actually why the Attendance Allowance is paid in the first place – to purchase the care that they need.

## Direct Payments Act 1997

The Direct Payments Act enables local authorities to make an assessment of the care needs of people aged under 65, and if they lack the financial resources themselves, provide them with the resources to purchase the care directly from a care provider. The provider of care may include a member of the family or a friend, provided they are not living in the same home and are not part of the 'household'. The payment cannot be used to purchase care from the local authority in-house service but may well result in an increase in demand for care services from the independent sector.

People assuming responsibility for the purchase of their own care, through the Direct Payments, may be unaware of their responsibilities as an employer of the carer, including health and safety issues and the need for liability insurance.

Implementation of the Act is still very variable across local authorities. *Modernising Social Services* proposes that the age limit be abolished and that Direct Payments be introduced for people aged 65 and over. The implications of this proposal for the provision and regulation of home care are still being considered.

The Age Concern Books' annual publication *Your Rights* (see p 244) gives detailed information on the money benefits to which older people may be entitled.

**In summary**  Most of the people you care for, apart from those on Income Support, will be expected to contribute towards the cost of the care provided which enables them to continue to live in their own homes. Where the care is purchased direct from a private agency and the local authority social services department is not involved, individuals will be meeting the full cost themselves.

## CASE STUDY

**Mr Y** lives alone in his own home. He is 77 years old and has had a stroke and is now confined to a wheelchair. The home care service agreed to visit three times a day to assist with washing and dressing, to encourage Mr Y to eat and to assist with toileting.

Mr Y has a large family. However, only one daughter is involved with his care. She collects his pension and attendance allowance and deals with all matters relating to finance. She also makes sure he has adequate supplies of clean clothing and enough food. Mr Y has meals-on-wheels and home care provided by a private agency on behalf of the local authority.

Within a short period of time it became obvious that Mr Y was being neglected. There was not enough food in the house, never any money left and not enough clean clothes. Eventually Mr Y's health deteriorated and this debts began to mount up. He owed money for the home care service, his television was repossessed and his gas was disconnected.

A care manager was introduced to the case and he arranged to speak to all family members who agreed that the Home Carer could manage Mr Y's finances and assist with budgeting.

In time, all the arrears were paid. Mr Y also had sufficient food and an adequate supply of clothing.

## QUESTIONS

1. If you were the Home Carer in this situation, what would you do to assist Mr Y manage his affairs?

2. What do you think would be the main issues of concern in relation to Mr Y's daughter?

## RELEVANT ORGANISATIONAL POLICIES AND GUIDELINES

■ Handling of money and finance

■ Accepting gifts/legacies from service users

■ Charging policy of the organisation and methods of collecting the charge

■ Confidentiality

## KEY POINTS

■ You need to be aware of the basis on which people are charged for the care service you provide.

■ People receiving care should be encouraged to take full responsibility for their own financial affairs.

■ You need to handle money on behalf of those you are caring for with the utmost care and caution. You should resist getting involved in their financial matters other than shopping, paying bills and collecting their pension.

■ The people you are caring for will look to you as a source of information on a wide range of financial matters, benefits and welfare rights. You need to know where to go to obtain the information they seek.

■ It is natural that the people you care for will wish to show their appreciation, but you should only ever accept small and modest gifts. To accept expensive gifts could be considered improper conduct. Not to accept small gifts could give offence.

■ Resist any suggestion that you should be mentioned in someone's Will and report it to your line manager.

■ Never mix your own finances and personal money with those of someone you are caring for.

**CHECKLIST – FINANCIAL MATTERS**

| Do | Do not |
|---|---|
| Keep client's money entirely separate from your own. | Mix up your own personal money with that of the person you are caring for. |
| Always keep a careful record of the money given to you. | Leave settling the account until the end of the week, when the person may have forgotten about the transactions. |
| Obtain receipts for the foods and anything else you buy on behalf of those you are caring for. | |

*Continued*

**CHECKLIST – FINANCIAL MATTERS**

| Do | Do not |
|---|---|
| Settle up the account as soon as possible. | Borrow money or anything else from people you are caring for or lend them money. |
| Itemise all the transactions and take the person through them carefully. | Buy from or sell anything to someone you are caring for. |
| Exercise strict confidentiality about everything you might know about someone else's financial affairs. | Accept gifts other than very small tokens such as chocolates or soap, etc, which might be exchanged at Christmas. |
| **Report to your line manager if:** | Talk about your own financial affairs. |
| Someone insists on giving you money as a mark of appreciation. | Suggest – even as a joke – that someone should remember you in their Will. |
| You are told that you are to be a beneficiary in the Will of someone you are caring/have cared for. | Ask anyone you care for to be a guarantor for a hire purchase application. |
| You are accused by the client/family/friends of stealing money or any other item, or any other dishonesty. | Tell anyone other than your line manager if you find large amounts of money in a person's home. |
| You think someone you are caring for is being the victim of dishonesty by a third person or persons. | |
| You find large amounts of cash about the home. | |

# 12 Terminal Illness and Death

S/NVQ Level 2: This chapter relates to the mandatory units 01, CL1 and Z1; Option Group A units W2, W3, Z19; Option Group B units CU3, Z8, Z16.

This chapter looks briefly at some of the points to note in providing home care to people who are terminally ill. This is skilled, specialist work which you should not be expected to undertake unless you have considerable experience of working as a Home Carer and have completed an appropriate training programme.

## Providing care for those who are terminally ill

Perhaps the most difficult thing you will be asked to do as a Home Carer will be to care for someone who is terminally ill. It is common for Home Carers to become very close to the people they are caring for, and coping with the long terminal illness of a friend can place stress and many pressures on you. On the other hand, the ill person will want to continue to receive care at home from people who they know and trust. They will not want to be looked after by strangers at this point in their lives, if it could possibly be avoided.

It is often very important to the dying person and their relatives that they are allowed to stay at home until the end. The increasing focus on hospital care for acute admissions will mean that people who are ill – but for whom there is no cure – will be cared for during their terminal illness in a residential home, a hospice, or in greater numbers, in their own home. It is therefore increasingly likely that Home Carers will be caring for people who are terminally ill and dying.

It is essential that care is provided with dignity and compassion. You will not be alone in providing care. It is probable that a qualified nursing specialist will be in charge and the care will be shared with others, including the person's own family and friends. Specialist services may be involved, such as Macmillan nurses and Marie Curie Cancer Care.

Caring for people who are terminally ill is skilled work. It is essential that a consistent approach is adopted. You should not find yourself being expected to provide care for people who are terminally ill without having been given in advance the necessary guidance, training and briefing on the particular individual situation. The home will need to be made suitable for providing the care necessary yet still retaining the home atmosphere – not turning the home into a hospital ward. Comfort may be given by physical care, including holding the person's hand and other appropriate touching, and listening and speaking in a calm manner.

Points to note for guidance:

- Everyone faces death differently. Do not make assumptions – treat every situation as unique.
- The aim should be to make the person as comfortable as possible – in mind as well as in body.
- Watch for symptoms of pain so that medical help can be summoned as often as necessary to ensure the person's continued comfort.
- In many cases, the person will know of their condition and may need to talk about it and their impending death. Most Home Carers are sympathetic listeners and can play an important role by helping people and their personal carers express fears about death and dying, and about other anxieties such as concern for those left behind. Talking about death should not be treated with embarrassment or brushed aside.

Family members often find it easier to talk about these issues and the situation to someone who is from outside the family. Think how you feel about talking to someone about death. If you think it will be difficult or distressing, talk to your line manager about it first.

**CHECKLIST – CARING FOR SOMEONE WHO IS TERMINALLY ILL**

■ The terminally ill person may wish to be involved in their own funeral arrangements. If they have no close family, you should be prepared to be involved in this process and to behave as naturally as possible.

■ If the person is **not** aware of their situation or the severity of their condition, you should **never** tell them.

■ You will need ready access to advice and guidance as the condition of the person deteriorates; for example, medical assistance in pain control and any other distressing symptoms of the illness.

■ The person you are caring for may very likely express a strong wish to remain at home. All concerned in the care of the person – including you – should do everything possible to comply with this wish. However, there will be occasions when this is just not possible.

■ The aim of all those involved in terminal care should be to make the life of the person as comfortable and fulfilling as possible.

■ There should be no forced jollity or contrived optimism, particularly if someone is aware of the eventual outcome of the condition. A simple open approach is best in helping the person to retain their dignity.

■ The preferences of the person and the family with regard to treatment, religious observance and cultural practices should be ascertained and carefully followed.

■ As death approaches, the person should not be left alone. Where requested by the person or their family, either at the time or before, the appropriate religious leader should be summoned.

■ News of the death should be given to the family, GP and others as soon as possible in a dignified manner.

■ Grief and mourning should not be hidden, but it should be accepted that some people may not openly display their emotions.

■ Staff who care for people who are dying are likely to be under considerable stress and need particular support. The problems of providing terminal care should be freely discussed among staff.

## Personal support

The work of a Home Carer can be emotionally rewarding but also very stressful.

If you are involved in providing care for people who are terminally ill, you should expect and, if necessary, request support from your line manager. Everyone involved in providing care for the dying person – family, friends and Home Carers – will need support, and perhaps counselling, after the death. This is perfectly natural.

You should also receive support if you experience the sudden death of a person you were caring for – particularly if you have looked after them for some time. Never underestimate the strain that the death of someone you care for will place on you.

**In summary** Do everything you can to assist yourself and others care for someone who is terminally ill and living in their own home. Ensure that you receive necessary training and support from your line manager.

## CASE STUDY

**Miss R** was a client in her 80s who lived alone in a large house which, although basically clean, was rather neglected. The garden, completely untended for many years, was gradually enclosing the house. Miss R had no next of kin but the home care service's contact was Miss M, who had known Miss R for over 50 years.

The Home Carers, who had visited Miss R over the last few years of her life, considered her eccentric. Those meeting her for the first time could consider her extremely rude, ignorant and awkward. Miss R was an animal lover, especially dogs. This was obvious from the old animal toys, dog leads, food dishes, etc, in the kitchen and the fact that crusts cut from sandwiches had to be kept for Miss M to feed the birds.

For the last three years of her life, Miss R was bedridden, her bed being in the living room. There were many books on shelves to the ceiling of this room, and it was obvious from their titles that Miss R was a very learned person. She was no longer able to read because of deteriorating vision. She had never had a television and would not use her radio because 'batteries are expensive'.

Miss R had four visits a day from the home care service: morning and lunch with one of the Home Carers, tea and late evening with two staff because of the very scary setting of her home. Towards the end, there were two Home Carers at all visits because of increasing dependency.

When more able, Miss R would see who the Home Carers were and 'choose' which one could stay in the room and see to her and which should be 'banished' to the kitchen. The first carer would assist Miss R to the commode and help with hygiene. The one in the kitchen would make coffee, using three grains of coffee, and scramble eggs (not runny) for breakfast. There were Marmite sandwiches for lunch and trifle made by Miss M and more Marmite sandwiches in the evening.

Miss R would shrink beneath her bed covers if anyone tried to give her any mail from the letter box, this had to be left in the hall for Miss M. The only exception to this was Christmas cards for which the Home Carer would be thanked. This may have been the only time Miss R ever spoke to a Home Carer if she was more familiar with their partner.

Incontinence pads had to be wrapped in several layers of newspaper before being put in the dustbin. For this task the Home Carer was allowed briefly to switch on the outside light.

After the visit, Miss R would ask the Home Carer to phone Miss M to make sure she was all right and to enquire after the health of her dog. They only ever addressed each other by Miss R and Miss M; never by first names.

When Miss R did not wish to take medication, she could eventually be persuaded 'just to shut you up'. She would allow the

Home Carer to dab at her hair with a brush for a few seconds, declaring 'that's fine'. Her hair resembled a bird's nest. She would also dab her face with a flannel and towel.

Miss R was reluctantly admitted to hospital where she refused to allow tests to be done.

She had a medical problem which caused her to become more and more anaemic and the end result was inevitable, but she wanted to die at home. Right up to this time her memory was incredible – she may have chosen not to speak to a Home Carer for some months, but if she decided to, she would ask after their family members by name or ask about something even they themselves may have forgotten telling her about.

For the last weeks of life, she faded slowly. The Home Carers did their utmost to ensure her wish to die at home was fulfilled. The Home Carers often spent more than the allocated paid time with her. They were so pleased for her that she got her wish. Just before she died she told one of the Home Carers 'Thank you for all that you have all done for me. I am very grateful.'

## QUESTIONS

1. What do you think would be the main issues involved in providing care to Miss R in her last days?

2. Who else do you think could have been involved in providing the care?

# KEY POINTS

■ Caring for people who are terminally ill is specialised and demanding work but can be very rewarding. There is likely to be an increase in the number of terminally ill people who will be cared for in their own homes.

■ As a Home Carer you will not be working on your own but as part of a team which includes specialist nursing and medical help as required, as well as the person's own family.

■ You will need to provide care with dignity and compassion.

■ The aim of the care is to make the remaining life of the dying person as comfortable and fulfilling as possible.

■ Following the death, all concerned will need help and support. Family and friends will be distressed and will often turn to the Home Carer for support, as someone outside of the family.

■ The Home Carer may be distressed and in need of support from their line manager and colleagues.

# *13* Taking Care of Yourself

**S/NVQ Level 2: This chapter relates to the mandatory units O1, CL, CU1, Z1.**

This final chapter considers what you can do to take care of yourself. It looks at what you wear to work and general health and safety implications. It also considers your personal health and how you should respond to the stress of the work.

The most important person in the home care service is the person for whom you are providing the care. The second most important person is you, the Home Carer.

The previous chapters of this book all focus on the service you provide. This chapter focuses on you, because without you, and many other people like you, there would be no home care service. As far as the person you are caring for is concerned – you *are* the service. You need to remember that you are representing the service at all times when you are at work.

You need to take care of yourself and adopt safe working practices at all times in order to be able to continue to provide the vital service that your customers depend upon. If you don't look after and care for yourself, you will not be able to provide care for others. If you are off sick it causes disruption to the people you are caring for and is a high cost to either you, if you are self-employed, or the organisation which employs you.

The aim of this chapter is to enable you to maintain a healthy and enjoyable lifestyle, whether you are at home, at work or at leisure.

The benefits to you are that you will be able to enjoy life to the full and be a valuable member of the team at work. If you look after yourself, this should increase your job satisfaction and improve your morale.

There are a number of different ways in which you can look after yourself in relation to your work as a Home Carer. Some of the most important of these are explored in the following paragraphs.

## Wearing the right clothes

It is important that you wear the right clothes, including shoes, when you are at work.

All employing agencies should provide you with protective clothing. This will include, at the very least, some form of overall and rubber gloves. Most agencies will provide a change of clothing to allow for washing. If insufficient or inadequate protective clothing is provided, this should be reported to your line manager.

Protective clothing is provided because it is necessary and should be worn whenever you undertake certain activities. Your employing organisation should provide you with guidance on those activities which require you to wear the protective clothing. You may also choose to wear it yourself when undertaking other activities. It is sensible to explain to the person you are caring for, why you are wearing the protective clothing so that you do not, unintentionally, cause your customer unnecessary anxiety.

The organisation you work for may provide you with a uniform to wear when you are at work. Opinion on this is divided. There are views for and against the wearing of uniforms. Before 1993, when most of the service was provided by local authority social services departments, few, if any, provided uniforms. Home Carers were allowed and encouraged to wear their own everyday clothes so that they did not appear 'official' and intimidating to the people receiving care, to emphasise the 'normality' of the service they provided and to differentiate Home Carers from district and community nurses.

However, many of the private and voluntary sector agencies do provide uniforms for their Home Carers and some local authorities are now doing the same so that Home Carers do not have to spend their own money on the purchase of clothes for work.

If you are providing your own clothes, make sure whatever you are wearing does not restrict your movement and is loose-fitting. Be aware that long, full skirts can cause you to trip and fall, particularly on stairs, and full, loose sleeves can catch on door handles, shelves, hooks, etc.

If you are providing services to people from ethnic minority communities, you should take their culture and beliefs into consideration and wear clothes that are culturally sensitive. This may mean covering your arms and chest and/or wearing a longer skirt than usual.

It is also not advisable in most circumstances to wear very fashionable or expensive clothes. They may get damaged and the people you are caring for may not appreciate them!

The same also applies to the wearing of jewellery. Rings may scratch furniture or even the person you are caring for if you are helping them get out of bed or a chair or providing them with personal care. Long necklaces can get caught on a range of household items. Even dangling earrings may be a hazard! Just think what you are going to be doing in your work, before you put on your jewellery.

Shoes can be another hazard. You will be on your feet for some hours. Therefore you will need to wear low-heeled, comfortable shoes. They will probably need to fit well. If your feet can easily slip out of your shoes, you may find they become a hazard on loose carpets or on stairs. Wearing 'flip flops' or Dr Scholls sandals is probably not a good idea in the circumstances! Nor is it a good idea to wear 'designer' shoes with platform soles or chunky high heels. These make moving and handling very dangerous indeed.

You need to be aware that if you have an accident caused by wearing unsuitable clothing or shoes, in contradiction of the policy of your employing organisation, you may not be covered by their insurance policy.

**In summary** In general, when you are working as a Home Carer, it is best to wear plain, simple clothes and very little jewellery. Always wear protective clothing when required.

# Health and safety

Chapter 7 on 'Health and Safety' identified your role and responsibility in relation to the legislation and the European Directive on manual handling and lifting. These laws and regulations have been passed for your safety as well as the safety of the people you are caring for. Therefore you should always take account of safe working practices at all times. This includes the wearing of protective clothing as identified above. Many agencies now also supply Home Carers with residual current devices (known as RCDs) or circuit breakers. These are to protect you from the danger of electric shock, as the wiring and electrical appliances in other people's homes may not be up to a safe standard. So just like the protective clothing – do use it. As the saying goes – it is better to be safe than sorry!

However, it is human nature to want to respond to a potentially hazardous situation when it arises. This may include moving a heavy or bulky object or assisting the person you are caring for out of a chair or bed. You should be aware of how to undertake these tasks safely, have received the appropriate training and know when to seek assistance.

Back strains and back problems are a common cause of illness and sick absence in the home care service. Failure to observe the health and safety requirements, however well intentioned, can prove very costly and inconvenient, not only for you but also for the people you are caring for and your employing organisation.

Before beginning to provide a home care service, a risk assessment must be undertaken, as well as an assessment of need. Your line manager or someone else in your employing organisation has a responsibility to undertake a risk assessment before you enter the home, but it should also have been done by the person responsible for assessing the need and commissioning the care package.

However, nothing stays still, and over a period of time the degree of risk may have changed as well as the care needs. For example, the person you are caring for may become less mobile or bed-bound and require a hoist. The electric circuit may start sparking or carpets become very worn and frayed or detached from the stairs. These and other similar situations require a reassessment of the risks involved in delivering the care, and should always be reported to your line manager for action.

**In summary** Do not take risks. Always follow safe working practice and health and safety guidelines. Tell your line manager if any change occurs in the risks involved in providing care.

# Your health in general

If you look after your own health, you will also be showing concern for the health of the people you are caring for. Many of them will be frail and in poor health. You need to be aware that a minor health problem that causes minimum inconvenience to you, may present a major health problem to someone who is more vulnerable because of their age, frailty or disability. For example a common cold, which we all get from time to time, should not prevent you from going to work, but you should consider wearing a face mask to ensure that you do not transfer any germs to the people you are caring for.

If in doubt as to the severity of your cold, seek the advice of your line manager. The danger of you passing on your cold to your customers will need to be considered against the difficulty in providing replacement cover.

It is worth considering having a regular health check, particularly if you are a woman, and taking advantage of those offered routinely, such as smear tests and mammograms. You should always ensure that inoculations are kept up to date. This includes tetanus, hepatitis and polio. You may also wish to consider having an annual 'flu jab' to protect you against catching a bout of influenza.

It is always sensible to eat plenty of fresh fruit and vegetables and to restrict consumption of fat, carbohydrates and alcohol. Taking regular exercise is also beneficial – but you may well feel that your work as a Home Carer provides you with more than enough exercise!

If you smoke, you should be aware of the effect this can have on others. Your employing organisation may have a policy on smoking on duty. Even if they haven't, it is good practise **not** to smoke whilst in someone else's house, even if they smoke themselves.

**In summary** Try to adopt a healthy lifestyle and way of living. This will help you in all aspects of your life, not only in your work.

# Harassment

Your employing organisation should have a policy on harassment which should provide guidelines for you to follow. Through training, you should also be familiar with your organisation's policy on equal opportunities and anti-discriminatory practice – or at the very least know where you can go to obtain the information.

The likelihood of harassment occurring may be reduced by matching Home Carers to the people needing care and/or sending two people together to the person's home. However, staff shortages and recruitment difficulties often make this hard to achieve in practice.

Harassment may take different forms. It is generally either verbal or physical, but it may be visual in the form of leaving offensive material around for the Home Carer to see. Whatever form the harassment takes, it is always nasty and offensive to the person who is being harassed. Only you can decide what you personally consider to be unacceptable behaviour. You may not wish to report the first incident of harassment to your line manager as it may be an isolated incident, but you should consider keeping a record and reporting it if such incidents persist.

Everyone has a right not to be discriminated against and this equally applies to Home Carers. It is not unknown for people receiving care and/or their family carers to make offensive remarks to Home Carers concerning the colour of their skin, religion, race or relating to sex. Whatever the nature of the offensive remark, it should never be condoned. You do not have to accept or put up with such bad behaviour, even if the person concerned is old and vulnerable – that is no excuse.

You need to be aware that some people may behave inappropriately and without any inhibitions as the result of illness such as dementia, or because of disability. You should discuss any such difficulties with your line manager.

You should also be aware that your own behaviour may encourage harassment. Over-familiarity in your way of speaking or your manner with the people you care for, and their family carers, particularly of the opposite sex, may be misinterpreted and lead to harassment. It is preferable to keep a distance between you and the people you care for. Be friendly at all times but not too familiar.

**In summary** You should never have to accept any form of harassment from the people you are caring for. It is unacceptable behaviour which you should record and report to your line manager.

# Handling aggression

It is possible, although thankfully it doesn't happen very often, that people you are caring for and/or their carers may become verbally or physically aggressive towards you. This is also often the result of illness and/or frustration with becoming old, infirm and dependent upon others. They may also be frightened about what is happening to them and express this in an aggressive way. You should be told at the very beginning if there is any possibility that any of the people you are caring for may become aggressive and violent. However, some people may deteriorate over time and become more aggressive as their condition deteriorates. Your line manager should be informed and a reassessment of need requested.

You should be provided with training by your employing authority on the possible causes of aggression and the way to handle such incidents. Training should provide you with ways of avoiding conflict and defusing difficult situations. However, the reality is that it is never easy and all occurrences of actual physical aggression should be reported to your line manager and an accident report form completed.

If at all possible, the potential of physical aggression should have been identified at the time that the original risk assessment was undertaken. As with harassment, the provision of two Home Carers should reduce the likelihood of physical attack.

**In summary** You should be informed of any potentially aggressive situations and receive training on avoiding conflict and defusing difficult situations.

# Working conditions

We have already considered in this book how home care has changed over the last five years. The provision of flexible services to meet the needs of people requiring care means an increase in work early in the morning to assist people getting out of bed and in the late evening to help them go to bed. There is also a growth in night checking services. Such unsocial hours of work make Home Carers more vulnerable to the danger of attack.

Your employing organisation should take all the necessary precautions to safeguard your safety as far as possible, whilst you are at work. This should include the provision of a bleep or alarm, ensuring appropriate transport is available and enabling Home Carers to work in pairs. Some organisations may provide a mobile telephone. You also need to take care that you do not expose yourself to unnecessary risk. Halogen lights fixed over the front or back door of the homes you are visiting at night may also increase your safety.

It is known that some Home Carers, because of the part-time nature of the work, work for more than one home care organisation. If you are in this position, you should be aware that the European Directive, which came into effect in 1998, stipulates the maximum number of hours you can work as 48 per week with mandatory break periods during the working day and days off. This is to protect your health and safeguard that of your customers who may suffer if you become over-tired or ill.

Your employer will not expect you to work in excessively hot or cold conditions. If the environment in the home is bad for you, it will almost certainly be even worse for the person you are caring for. If you were working in an office and the temperature reached an unacceptable level, your employer would send you home. Unfortunately, that does not apply to work in people's own homes, and all you can do is to notify your line manager as to the conditions in which you are working and ensure they take action including a reassessment of need and risk assessment if necessary.

**In summary** Your employer should take all reasonable precautions to protect your safety when working unsocial hours. However, you should not expose yourself to any unnecessary risk.

# Stress

Providing home care is a very demanding, yet rewarding job. Many Home Carers become close to the people they are caring for, often over a number of years. This may lead to them undertaking more tasks, out of work hours. Over time this builds up and increases the stress and strain of the work. The opportunity to have regular supervision sessions with your line manager can help explore the issues and monitor the stress you are experiencing.

The death of someone you were caring for can be very stressful, particularly if you have been caring for them for a considerable length of time. You will need time to grieve and recover from your loss. If you loose more than one customer in a short space of time, this will increase the pressure and stress placed upon you.

In these circumstances you should seek the assistance and support of your line manager who should provide you with time to talk the matter through. The provision of regular one-to-one supervision should assist you cope with the stress and help your line manager to monitor the situation. You may also find your colleagues are a great comfort, most, if not all of whom will have had similar experiences.

**In summary** Recognise the stress that the work creates. Take what steps you can to reduce it and seek help and support from your line manager.

## RELEVANT ORGANISATIONAL POLICIES AND GUIDELINES

■ When protective clothing must be worn

■ Dress code (including guidelines on uniforms if provided)

■ Health and safety policy

■ Smoking and drinking alcohol while at work

■ Equal opportunities and anti-discriminatory practice

■ Harassment – sexual and racial

■ Handling aggression

■ Working conditions, including out of hours

■ Emergency procedures

## CASE STUDY

**Mrs P** is in her late 60s and has suffered a series of strokes which have left her with considerable residual paralysis and unable to communicate verbally. Her husband is her main carer and he insists on interpreting Mrs P's wishes. An intensive domiciliary care package is in place and there is mixed provision from both the public and private sector.

A manual handling risk assessment has been undertaken and Mrs P has been assessed as needing two people to move her using a hoist when she needs to move from the bed to the commode. The staff have been advised on the most appropriate techniques and Mr P has been fully briefed on the correct moving and handling arrangements for his wife.

Mr P is unhappy that the staff are not able to lift his wife and, taking advantage of his wife's inability to communicate, set about convincing certain individuals that Mrs P is distressed about the use of the hoist. Several Home Carers were sympathetic to Mr P's views and, ignoring their instructions to use the hoist, began to lift Mrs P. Mr P then used this as an opportunity to play one member of staff off against the other, causing serious conflict between the Home Carers and their respective employers.

These unfortunate events resulted in three Home Carers reporting sick. Two were suffering from stress caused by the bad feelings as the work group became divided and one had a back injury through lifting Mrs P.

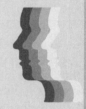

## QUESTIONS

If you were faced with this situation, how would you respond, and what action would you take in respect of:

1. Mrs P?

2. Mr P?

3. Your fellow Home Carers?

4. Your employer?

**CHECKLIST –TAKING CARE OF YOURSELF**

| Do | Do not |
|---|---|
| Wear the protective clothing provided whenever required. | Wear long, flowing skirts or other clothes which may cause you to trip or get caught on door handles, etc. |
| Wear low-heeled, comfortable shoes that will not slip. | |
| Wear plain, inexpensive clothes. | Take unnecessary risks such as lifting heavy weights or bulky objects on your own. |
| Observe all health and safety procedures and guidelines. | |
| Use an RCD if provided and available. | Expose your customers to the danger of catching your cold. |
| Have a regular health check and keep inoculations up to date. | Smoke cigarettes in the homes of your customers. |
| Eat healthily and take plenty of exercise. | Do anything to encourage harassment or an aggressive response. |
| Take appropriate precautions if you have a cold. | Be over-familiar in your words or actions. |
| Report incidents of harassment and aggression to your line manager. | Expose yourself unnecessarily to risk of attack when working unsocial hours, eg late at night. |
| Ensure you are equipped with alarms or a bleep. | Wear rings or jewellery which can catch on furniture or scratch. |

# APPENDIX 1

# S/NVQ in Care Level 2

To gain this award, a candidate must achieve all four mandatory units, plus five option units (at least three of which must be chosen from Option Group A).

## Mandatory units

O1      Foster people's equality, diversity and rights

CL1     Promote effective communication and relationships

CU1     Promote, monitor and maintain health, safety and security in the workplace

Z1      Contribute to the protection of individuals from abuse

### OPTION GROUP A

CL2     Promote communication with individuals where there are communication differences

CU5     Receive, transmit, store and retrieve information

NC12    Enable clients to eat and drink

W2      Contribute to the ongoing support of clients and others significant to them

W3      Support individuals experiencing a change in their care requirements

Z6      Enable clients to maintain and improve their mobility through exercise and the use of mobility appliances

Z7      Contribute to the movement and treatment of clients to maximise their physical comfort

Z9      Enable clients to maintain their personal hygiene and appearance

Z11     Enable clients to access and use toilet facilities

**Z19**   Assist clients to achieve physical comfort

## OPTION GROUP B

**CL5**   Promote communication with those who do not use a recognised language format

**CU3**   Monitor and maintain the cleanliness of environments

**CU4**   Support and control visitors to services and facilities

**CU6**   Assist in supplying and maintaining materials and equipment

**CU10**   Contribute to the effectiveness of work teams

**NC13**   Prepare food and drink for individual clients

**W6**   Reinforce professional advice through supporting and encouraging the mother in active parenting in the first ten days of babies' lives

**W8**   Enable clients to maintain contacts in potentially isolating situations

**X1**   Contribute to the support of clients during development programmes and activities

**Y1**   Enable clients to manage their domestic and personal resources

**Z5**   Enable clients to maintain their mobility and make journeys and visits

**Z8**   Support clients when they are distressed

**Z13**   Enable clients to participate in recreation and leisure activities

**Z15**   Contribute to the care of a deceased person

**Z16**   Care for a baby in the first ten days of life when the mother is unable

# APPENDIX 2

# S/NVQ in Care Level 2 Unit O1

## UNIT O1 Foster people's equality, diversity and rights

### Elements of competence

O1.1   Foster people's rights and responsibilities

O1.2   Foster equality and diversity of people

O1.3   Maintain the confidentiality of information

### Information about this unit

SUMMARY

This unit is about acknowledging the equality and diversity of people and their rights and responsibilities. Due to the often sensitive nature of the information about people with which the sector deals, the maintenance of confidentiality is also included. Whilst it is recognised that workers are not always in a position to change and influence structures directly, they are expected to be proactive against discrimination.

The standards recognise that to acknowledge people's equality, diversity and rights, the worker has to be able to handle a number of competing tensions: within people themselves and between different people. Discrimination against people may occur for a wide range of reasons such as: differing abilities, age, class, caste, creed, culture, gender, health status, relationship status, mental health, offending background, place of origin, political beliefs, race, responsibility for dependants, religion, sexuality.

The term 'people' is used broadly to cover individuals, families, groups, communities and organisations. The people may be clients, colleagues or anyone else with whom the worker comes into contact.

WHO THIS UNIT IS AIMED AT

The unit is designed to be applicable to anyone who works in the health and social care sector and whose work role is limited in terms of accountability or overall responsibility, generally those who work in a supporting role to others.

## *O1.1  Foster people's rights and responsibilities*

PERFORMANCE CRITERIA

(1) The worker's actions recognise people's right to make their own decisions and acknowledge their responsibilities

(2) The worker's actions in interpreting the meaning of rights and responsibilities are consistent with existing legislative frameworks and organisational policy

(3) **Information** provided by the worker is up-to-date and takes account of the complexity of the decisions which people may need to make

(4) People who are unable to exercise their rights personally are given the **appropriate help** to do so

(5) **Tensions** between rights and responsibilities are acknowledged and the **appropriate support** is given towards their resolution

(6) The necessary records relating to the promotion of rights and responsibilities are accurate, legible and complete

(7) People who wish to make a complaint about an infringement of their rights are provided with the necessary information to do so

RANGE

1 **Information:**

a) verbal

b) written

2 **Appropriate help to exercise rights:**

a) speaking on behalf of the person when they are not able to do so

b) seeking support from someone else to help in the exercise of rights

3 **Tensions:**

a) within people

b) between people

4 **Appropriate support towards resolution:**

a) direct challenges to the people concerned

b) help sought from others towards a resolution

## O1.2 Foster equality and diversity of people

PERFORMANCE CRITERIA

(1) Actions of the worker are consistent with people's expressed beliefs and views and acknowledge the benefits of **diversity**

(2) Anti-discriminatory practice is promoted in ways which are consistent with legislative frameworks and organisational policy

(3) The **appropriate action** is taken to minimise the impact of discrimination and oppression on people

(4) Advice and guidance are sought by the worker when they are having difficulty promoting equality and diversity

(5) Information recorded by the worker is consistent with the promotion of equality and diversity

RANGE

1 **Diversity:**

a) individual and social characteristics

b) values and beliefs

2 **Appropriate action:**

a) challenge the source of the discrimination

b) seek the support of others to challenge

## NOTES ON THIS ELEMENT

In range statement (1): (a) individual and social characteristics: will include age, gender, sexuality, place of origin, race, health status, abilities, class, caste, relationship status, offending background, responsibility for dependants; (b) values and beliefs will include: creed, culture, political beliefs, religion.

## O1.3 Maintain the confidentiality of information

### PERFORMANCE CRITERIA

(1)  **Information stored** in, and retrieved from, recording systems is consistent with the requirements of legislation and organisational policy

(2)  Records made by the worker are accurate and legible and only contain the information necessary for the record's purpose

(3)  Information is only disclosed to those who have the right and need to know once proof of identity has been obtained

(4)  The **appropriate precautions** are taken when **communicating** confidential or sensitive information to those who have the right and need to know it

(5)  When someone tells the worker something which the worker is required to share with others, the person is clearly told in an appropriate manner that the information **will be shared with others**

(6)  Confidential records are handled securely and stored in the correct place

### RANGE

1  **Information stored:**

  a) electronically

  b) in writing

2  **Appropriate precautions in relation to:**

  a) who might overhear or oversee the information

  b) who might access the information

## 3 Communicating:

a) electronically

b) in writing

c) orally

## NOTES ON THIS ELEMENT

'Appropriate precautions' in performance criterion (4) will depend on a number of factors such as: how the information is being communicated, the setting, who else is or may be present, who else accesses the setting at other times.

'Information which the worker is required to share' in performance criterion (5) might include: indicators that the health and social well-being of the person who told the worker is at risk, others may be put at risk, the person is indicating symptoms of ill health which need to be acted on and are in their plan of care (eg hearing voices), indicators of abuse, information which directly affects the organisation and its effectiveness. Such requirements may be identified in places as: codes of conduct, plans of care, legislation.

# APPENDIX 3

## Chapters of *CareFully* related to S/NVQ units in Care Level 2

This book provides underpinning knowledge and information to cover all the units required to achieve a Level 2 award in Care.

| Chapter | Title | Mandatory Units | Optional Units A | Optional Units B |
|---------|-------|-----------------|------------------|------------------|
| 1 | Receiving Home Care | O1, CL1 | | |
| 2 | The Importance of Core Values | O1, CL1, CU1, Z1 | | |
| 3 | Providing a Service for the New Millennium | *O1, CL1* | *CU5, W2, W3* | |
| 4 | The Health of Older People | O1, CL1, Z1 | W2, W3, Z7, Z9, Z19 | CU3, W8, Y1, Z8 |
| 5 | Making the First Contact | O1, CL1, Z1 | *CU5, W2* | W8, Y1, |
| 6 | The Basic Skills of Home Carers | O1, CL1, CU1, Z1 | *CU5, W2* | CU3, W8, Y1, |
| 7 | Health and Safety | O1, CL1, CU1, Z1 | Z9, Z11, Z19, W2 | *CU3, Y1* |
| 8 | Eating and Nutrition | O1, CL1, Z1 | *NC12, W2* | CU3, NC13, Y1 |
| 9 | Mobility and Disability | O1, CL1, CU1, Z1 | Z6, Z7, Z9, Z11, Z19, W2 | *Y1, Z5* |
| 10 | Maintaining Continence | O1, CL1, Z1 | Z7, Z9, Z11, Z19, W2 | *CU3, Z8* |
| 11 | Financial Matters | O1, CL1, Z1 | *W2* | *Y1* |
| 12 | Terminal Illness and Death | O1, CL1, Z1 | W2, W3, Z19 | CU3, Z8, Z16 |
| 13 | Taking Care of Yourself | O1, CL1, CU1, Z1 | | |

# APPENDIX 4

# Policies and Practices of the Organisation

The Home Carer works in difficult, challenging and generally isolated circumstances. You therefore need all the help and assistance you can get, and it is unreasonable for any employing agency to expect you to work in a vacuum.

The employing agency should itself provide a basis and a framework for the provision of home care by supplying the following information on the organisation's policies and practices to every Home Carer.

You may like to place a tick alongside those you have copies of:

- Aims and objectives of the organisation.
- Conditions of employment, including travel expenses and rights to join a trade union.
- Contract of employment and job description, including the activities required to be undertaken.
- Clarification of activities you are *not* supposed to undertake.
- Personal safety and out-of-hours working.
- Standards you are expected to maintain in your work and means of assuring the standards.
- Information on the care plan for each service user (if compiled); alternatively, information on (assessed) care needs of each service user.
- The provision of non-discriminatory practice.
- Equal opportunities and sexual harassment.
- Complaints procedure.
- Confidentiality of information.
- Health and safety regulations, including accident report procedure.
- What action to take in an emergency.
- Dress code, including protective clothing.
- Data protection and subject access.
- Charging policy of the organisation.
- Handling and administering medicines.

■ Moving and handling.
■ Handling money and finance (on behalf of people receiving care).
■ Accepting gifts/legacies from service users.
■ Safe keeping of keys.
■ Handling violence and aggression.
■ Harassment – sexual and racial.
■ Smoking and drinking at work.

It is unreasonable and irresponsible of any employing organisation to expect any of their Home Carers to undertake their work efficiently and effectively without such basic information and 'ground rules'.

# APPENDIX 5

# Issues or Situations to be Referred to Others for Guidance or Action

The following occurrences or situations, which are referrred to in the related chapter, should always be discussed or reported to the appropriate person – generally your line manager or the manager of your employment agency.

### Chapter 2 The Importance of Core Values

■ If you are concerned for the health, safety or welfare of the person you are caring for and may need to breech confidentiality.

### Chapter 3 Providing a Service for the New Millennium

■ When assessment (or reassessment) of care need is required.
■ If one of your customers wishes to make a formal complaint.

### Chapter 4 The Health of Older People

■ If you have any concern for the mental or physical condition of the person you are caring for.
■ If you need to contact the GP or local pharmacist about a person's medication.
■ Any medication which has passed its 'use by' date.
■ Any matter that could amount to physical or mental abuse of the person you are caring for.
■ Any concern about the sexual or uninhibited behaviour of a person you are caring for including sexual harassment.

### Chapter 5 Making the First Contact

■ If you are not provided with all the basic information you need before starting work with a new person, eg the care plan and the risk assessment.
■ Any conflict that arises between the tasks you are there to undertake as part of the care plan and those that the person you are caring for and/or their family carers want you to do.

■ Information on the standards to which you should work and any quality assurance measures that should be applied.

■ Training needs arising from the provision of services to people from ethnic minority communities.

■ The absence of written information in the home on points of contact for the service and in the case of an emergency.

## Chapter 6  The Basic Skills of Home Carers

■ Any issues in delivering complex packages of care.

■ Problems relating to a person smoking.

■ If you think the pattern of service delivery is causing any distress to the person receiving care.

## Chapter 7  Health and Safety

■ All accidents and other incidents.

■ Any new or potential health and safety risks or hazards.

■ If the fabric of the building is in need of repair and it is rented accommodation.

■ Any signs of pests and infestations.

■ Requests to assist with medication and administering ointment.

■ People who refuse to take a bath or shower.

■ People who refuse to use lifts or hoists or any defects in the equipment.

## Chapter 8  Eating and Nutrition

■ If a person is on a medical diet and insists on eating foods which are not recommended.

■ If you are unsure about what food to purchase and prepare to meet religious requirements or the needs of vegetarians and vegans.

■ Means of assisting people who are visually impaired, with their food.

■ If you are concerned about the possibility of alcohol abuse.

■ Provision of equipment and utensils which will enable someone with disabilities to feed themselves.

■ If a person refuses to eat.

## Chapter 9  Mobility and Disability

■ If you think there may be a need for aids and adaptations to assist mobility.

■ Signs of pressure sores.

## Chapter 10 Maintaining Continence

- If you suspect the onset of incontinence and the person you are caring for takes no action themselves.

## Chapter 11 Financial Matters

- If the person you are caring for wants you to collect their pension on their behalf.
- Any request to undertake more than basic financial transactions on behalf of anyone you are caring for.
- If you are concerned about valuables lying around the home.
- Any concern that the person is becoming confused and therefore unable to take care and responsibility for their own finances.

### Report to your line manager if:

- Someone insists on giving you money as a mark of appreciation.
- You are told that you are to be a beneficiary in the Will of someone you are caring/have cared for.
- You are accused by the client/family/friends of stealing money or any other item, or any other dishonesty.
- You think someone you are caring for is being the victim of dishonesty by a third person or persons.
- You find large amounts of cash about the home.

## Chapter 12 Terminal Illness and Death

- You need personal support when caring for someone with a terminal illness, or in the (unexpected) death of someone you have cared for, for some time.

## Chapter 13 Taking Care of Yourself

- Lack of adequate protective clothing.
- When a new risk assessment is required.
- If someone behaves in an uninhibited way or becomes aggressive.
- Any form of harassment.
- When feeling the effects of stress.

# APPENDIX 6

# Good Practice in Home Care

## Chapter 1  Receiving Home Care

■ Put yourself in the place of the person you are caring for and think how you would feel receiving care, and how you would wish to be treated.
■ Treat each person as an individual.
■ Consider the particular needs of personal and family carers.
■ Take time to establish an effective means of communication.
■ Establish at the beginning how the person wishes to be addressed by you.

## Chapter 2  The Importance of Core Values

■ Put into practice the principles which should underpin the provision of care to people in their own homes.
■ Ensure that you maintain confidentiality of personal information about the people you are caring for and never gossip about them to colleague Home Carers.
■ Ensure that you observe the rights of people who receive home care.
■ Always treat all the people you are caring for in exactly the same way as you would wish to be treated yourself.
■ Only work with people from ethnic minority communities when you have received the necessary training on the religious and cultural implications of providing care.

## Chapter 3  Providing a Service for the New Millennium

■ In the new millennium there will be national standards for regulating providers of home care and accrediting and registering care workers.
■ The services you provide are designed to meet the specific and individual needs of the people you are caring for.
■ People you care for and their families should be involved in decisions about the way in which their care needs will be met.
■ Ensure all the people you care for have copies of the complaints procedure in a suitable format, eg language, tape, braille.

■ Ensure that you receive all the training necessary to enable you to carry out your work to the expected standard. Work towards obtaining the S/NVQ Level 2 in Care.

## Chapter 4  The Health of Older People

■ Do all you can to encourage older people to seek help for medical and health problems – never assume that getting older automatically makes someone ill or disabled.

■ Always treat people according to their condition and not their age.

■ Pay as much attention to the person's emotional and social care as to their physical care and take what action you can to reduce isolation.

■ Note any physical or mental changes over time which might indicate deterioration in health and report to your line manager.

■ Be sure you know how to treat symptoms of hypothermia.

■ Ensure you observe safe working practices in the administration of medication.

■ If there is danger of physical attack or aggression, two Home Carers should be present.

■ Recognise the need everyone has for emotional fulfilment and social relationships, and behave and respond appropriately in each separate and different situation.

■ Be careful about the signals you give. Don't joke about sexual matters or make suggestive comments. Your motives may be misunderstood.

## Chapter 5  Making the First Contact

■ Ensure you have all the basic information you need about the person you are caring for and their needs.

■ Ensure the person you are caring for has all the necessary written information relating to their care plan, the service provider, who to contact in an emergency and the complaints procedure.

■ Your first visit to the home should be planned and structured, and follow an agreed procedure.

■ Learn as much as you can about the person's wants, needs and preferences from any family carers.

■ Recognise that the wants and needs of the family carer are separate and different from those of the person needing care.

■ As far as possible, arrange for your visits to take place at a different time to that of others involved in providing care – it helps to break up the day.

- Wherever possible, Home Carers should be 'matched' to the people they are caring for.
- Follow the agreed procedures on the holding of keys.
- Ensure there is a checklist in the home, displayed in a prominent place, with the name and address of key people to contact if necessary.

## Chapter 6 The Basic Skills of Home Carers

- Always arrive at the home on time
- On arrival at the home, enquire whether there is anything in particular the person would like done – and if possible and reasonable, do it.
- If there is a log in the home, check any comments left by other carers and keep it up to date.
- Always encourage the person to do some of the work with you. Avoid making them dependent.
- Always be aware that you are working in someone else's home and treat it accordingly.
- Respect the person's home and possessions. Treat them with care.
- Never smoke while in someone else's home and don't eat or drink unless specifically invited to do so.
- Support and maintain the person's independence as far as possible. Encourage them to do as much as possible for themselves.
- Do not impose your standards on the person you are caring for. Obtain permission before making changes in the home.
- Undertake the basic activities, taking account of the need to apply good caring skills.
- Know and recognise when situations give cause for concern and report them to the appropriate person.

## Chapter 7 Health and Safety

- Always adopt safe working practices. Identify potential hazards to the safety of the person as well as to yourself.
- Be aware of the need for hygienic working practices and wear protective clothing and rubber gloves.
- Always use your RCD.
- Identify possible hazards in the home and try to persuade the person to take appropriate action.
- Ensure that you receive training in moving and handling techniques, but never try to lift people or bulky and heavy objects yourself.

- Be familiar with the correct emergency procedures in a variety of situations.
- Have first-aid training.
- Take all appropriate precautions to secure the home.
- Recognise when a home is becoming insanitary and/or infested.
- Report all accidents.

## Chapter 8  Eating and Nutrition

- Recognise the importance of food and mealtimes, particularly for people who are housebound.
- Provide advice on healthy eating, a balanced diet and nutrition.
- Always observe strict hygiene precautions when handling food.
- People should always choose what they want to eat. They should also be involved as much as possible in shopping and in cooking and preparing food.
- Seek advice on the availability of special equipment and aids that make it easier for people with disabilities to prepare food, open cans and feed themselves (for example).
- Encourage and support people who are on special diets for medical or other reasons.
- Take time with people while they are eating their meal; provide any assistance necessary as requested by them.

## Chapter 9  Mobility and Disability

- Mobility is essential to maintain independence. Find appropriate ways of encouraging people to be as mobile as possible.
- Recognise the importance of exercise in maintaining the health of people you are caring for.
- Encourage people and their family carers to take care of the feet and to wear properly fitting shoes rather than slippers.
- Know where to go for information on aids and equipment to assist mobility.

## Chapter 10  Maintaining Continence

- Deal with matters relating to incontinence with great sensitivity.
- Recognise that incontinence can frequently be cured or at least improved, and encourage the person and/or their family carer to seek help and advice.

■ Assist the person to maintain a positive continence programme.

## Chapter 11  Financial Matters

■ Be able to refer the person to the appropriate agency to get financial advice.

■ Always clarify with the person exactly how much of their money you have spent and always give them receipts.

■ Always keep the person's money entirely separate from your own.

■ Never accept gifts from the person you are caring for.

■ Be aware of the basis of charging for the service you provide and recognise that the service user has a right to a full explanation of the costs.

## Chapter 12  Terminal Illness and Death

■ You should not be asked to provide care for someone who is terminally ill unless you are experienced as a Home Care Assistant and have received the appropriate training.

■ You will work as part of a team which will include family, friends and professional medical staff such as the district or community nurse.

■ You need to recognise the personal stress that such work will cause, and seek support from your line manager and colleagues.

## Chapter 13  Taking Care of Yourself

■ Take care of yourself so that you are both physically and mentally capable of caring for those who need your services.

■ Wear appropriate clothing, including suitable shoes and the uniform if supplied.

■ Do not wear jewellery that can catch on things and scratch.

■ Observe all the rules of health and safety, including manual handling to avoid back strains and problems.

■ Keep all your injections (eg tetanus) up to date and have a regular health check.

■ Do not expose yourself to any unnecessary risk of harassment, aggression or violence.

■ Be aware of the danger of stress and take steps to ensure that it does not affect you.

# APPENDIX 7

# Some Common Illnesses and Disabilities of Later Life

**Alcohol abuse** This can be a lifelong habit or start in retirement. Older alcohol abusers may fall frequently and become confused, incontinent or malnourished. They may become isolated and lonely if friends and family avoid them when they are unpleasant after drinking.

*Outlook* No one can be compelled to stop drinking; people who have done so to excess all their lives rarely change their behaviour in old age. All carers can do is try to reduce the dangers of and damage from their chosen lifestyle in whatever ways they can. People who 'take to drink' in later life can sometimes be helped, and may control their drinking if their health and social circumstances are improved.

**Alzheimer's disease** This is a form of dementia, a degenerative disease of the brain. Usually it is noticed in someone around the age of 80, and the cause is not known. A few of the rare cases that start before the age of 60 show an inherited pattern.

*Outlook* People with Alzheimer's disease do not get better and usually get worse, though how fast this happens varies from one person to another. There is no cure for the disease, but good medical care helps to control symptoms and to keep the sufferer as well as possible.

**Arthritis** There are several forms of this joint disease; the commonest is osteoarthritis (OA). Pain, stiffness and reduced mobility can be helped by: pain-relieving medicines; a balance of rest and exercise; warmth, as from a heating pad; and assessment by an occupational therapist and provision of equipment; physiotherapy; surgery to replace affected joints.

*Outlook* Arthritis is a painful nuisance but does not shorten life and only rarely becomes severe enough to interfere with independent living.

**Angina (pectoris)** Angina is a tight, squeezing chest pain caused by narrowing of the coronary arteries that supply the heart with blood. The pain may be brought on by exertion or emotion and is relieved by rest and pre-scribed medicines.

*Outlook* People with angina are at increased risk of suffering a heart attack. However, they can be helped by treatment and should be encour-aged to keep as active as possible within the limits of their pain.

**Breathing problems** These can be due to chronic bronchitis, emphysema or asthma in any combination. Some people are severely disabled by breathlessness all the year round, whilst others become much worse in the winter because of chest infections.

*Outlook* This depends on the severity of the condition. Stopping smok-ing will always help, and it is never too late to do so. Chest infections need prompt treatment with antibiotics; a 'chesty' person whose spit becomes green or yellow needs to see the doctor urgently.

**Brittle bones (osteoporosis)** The bones become weaker as the years pass, especially in women after the menopause. The softened vertebrae in the spine may become squashed, causing pain and stooping. Weakened hip and wrist bones may break easily.

*Outlook* Osteoporosis is not in itself dangerous, though it reduces inde-pendence and enjoyment of life. Some people who break their hips die of complications. Hormone replacement therapy helps to prevent osteo-porosis in women.

**Cancer** This happens when body cells multiply rapidly to form a tumour. Some cancers are said to be 'malignant' because they spread rapidly to other organs, causing serious disease and death. Others spread more slowly, and a person can live for years with them before dying of something else.

*Outlook* Very variable, depending on the type of cancer. Early diagnosis is important because early treatment may slow spread or even give a com-plete cure. Treatment can be by surgery, radiotherapy or drugs in any combination; though effective in the long run, this can cause serious unwanted effects in the short term. Advanced cancer can cause severe symptoms such as pain or breathlessness, and special skills of a hospice outreach team or a Macmillan nurse may be needed to keep the sufferer comfortable.

**Dementia** The dementias are a group of degenerative diseases of the brain, causing gradual loss of intellectual abilities and emotional skills. The commonest types are Alzheimer's disease and multi-infarct dementia, a form of stroke illness.

*Outlook* People with dementia get worse as time passes, though the rate of decline varies from person to person. It is important to make sure that the symptoms are not due to a curable physical illness. There is no medical cure for dementia. Good general care can greatly improve the sufferer's quality of life, and respite care may relieve relatives and help them to go on caring.

**Diabetes** In this condition the body is unable to process sugar properly because insulin is in short supply or the body has become insensitive to it. Older people usually develop a type of diabetes that can be controlled by diet and tablets without the need for insulin injections.

*Outlook* Complications can cause disability from heart, blood vessel and kidney disorders. Sight can deteriorate, and unnoticed and untreated skin ulcers lead to gangrene. Good control of diabetes makes these complications less likely, so you should encourage your clients to follow their treatment plans carefully. Regular eye checks and skilled chiropody are especially important.

**Hearing problems** These have many causes and should never be attributed to normal ageing; full assessment is required.

*Outlook* This depends on the cause. Medication may be helpful, and the person should be given advice and equipment to help them make the most of their remaining hearing.

**HIV/AIDS** The Human Immunodeficency Virus (HIV) is passed from one person to another in infected body fluids. This usually involves unprotected sex, use of contaminated injection equipment or passage of the virus from mother to baby before or during birth. The risks to those caring for people with AIDS are very small.

*Outlook* People who are positive for HIV develop the illnesses that form the AIDS complex, the Acquired Immunodeficiency Syndrome. Many of these happen because the person's resistance to infection is low. Eventually these illnesses prove fatal.

**Hypothermia** This is the condition in which central body temperature is low. Older people are vulnerable because their body's ability to control temperature deteriorates. Especially at risk are those who: have mobility problems or a tendency to fall; abuse alcohol; are mentally ill or mentally frail; are on low incomes; are isolated, with few visitors. With hypothermia, a person becomes sleepy and confused and a covered part of the body such as the armpit or abdomen feels cold to the touch. (For how to help, see pp 71–72.)

*Outlook* This depends on the circumstances; it is worse if the person has a severe underlying illness or has become very cold.

**Malnutrition** This can be caused by lack of teeth, by poor diet because of deficiency in shopping and cooking or lack of money, or by illnesses that interfere with the digestion and absorption of food.

*Outlook* This depends on the cause, which should be identified and put right whenever possible. Vitamins and other food supplements are sometimes necessary as a last resort.

**Mental health problems** Common ones in later life include depression, dementia (see above) and paranoid states. People with *depressive disorder* are preoccupied by gloomy thoughts, have no enjoyment of life and feel hopeless about the future. They may be slowed down and apathetic, or overactive and constantly seeking reassurance. They may complain of physical symptoms such as headache or abdominal pain but no physical explanation can be found. They are at risk from self-neglect or from deliberate self-harm: you should *always* report a client's suicidal thoughts to the doctor and/or your line manager.

*Outlook* People with depressive disorder can be helped by medical treatment, by psychotherapy and by improvement in their health and social circumstances. It is often overlooked in older people, so you should watch out for the signs.

**Paranoid states** People with paranoid states wrongly believe that others are a threat to them or their property. They become very anxious and may try to retaliate to their imagined injuries. Many people with this problem lead solitary lives and have problems with sight and hearing; they commonly suffer with tinnitus (noises in the ear).

*Outlook* Treatment is often helpful, but it may be difficult to get the patient to accept it. The community psychiatric nurse is often helpful in persuading the sufferer to have the treatment and in giving advice and support to carers.

**Parkinson's disease** This is a disorder of the nervous system, and affects the ability to move. Older sufferers complain mainly of stiffness and difficulty in moving about and walking, while tremor is more pronounced in younger people.

*Outlook* Medicines can be very helpful, but must always be taken exactly as prescribed; treatment may need to be adjusted by a specialist from time to time. Changing meal times or giving vitamins may interfere with the actions of drugs and make the person ill. Physiotherapy and speech therapy are sometimes helpful. Some Parkinson's sufferers develop a form of dementia.

**Sight problems** These have many causes and should never be attributed to normal ageing; full assessment is required.

*Outlook* This depends on the cause. Surgery and/or medicines may be helpful, and the person should be given advice and equipment to help them make the most of remaining sight.

**Strokes** These happen when part of the brain loses its blood supply. They can be minor, moderately severe or massive and fatal. Multi-infarct dementia is the result of a series of small strokes.

*Outlook* This depends on how badly the brain is damaged, how well the person is rehabilitated and whether they have other disabilities that will limit recovery. The effect on the person depends on which parts of the brain are damaged and how badly: one common problem is of weakness and loss of feeling down one side of the body, loss of vision to that side and sometimes difficulty in speaking or in understanding what is said.

# APPENDIX 8

# Sources of Further Information

## Action on Elder Abuse
1268 London Road
London SW16 4ER
Tel: 0181-764 7648

Elder Abuse Response Line: 0800 7314141 (10 am–4.30 pm, weekdays)

Aims to prevent abuse of older people by raising awareness, education, promoting research and the collection and dissemination of information. Action on Elder Abuse operates the Elder Abuse Response, which is a confidential helpline service providing information for anyone and emotional support for those involved.

## Alzheimer's Disease Society
2nd Floor
Gordon House
10 Greencoat Place
London SW1P 1PH
Tel: 0171-306 0606

Information, support and advice about caring for someone with Alzheimer's disease.

## Arthritis Care
18 Stephenson Way
London NW1 2HD
Tel: 0171-916 1500
Fax: 0171-916 1505
Freephone: 0800 289170 (Mon–Fri, 12 noon–4 pm)

Advice about living with arthritis, loan of equipment, holiday centres. Local branches in many areas.

## Association for Continence Advice
Winchester House
Kennington Park
Cranmer Road
London SW9 6EJ
Tel: 0171-820 8113
Fax: 0171-820 0442

Working on behalf of continence advisers, both nationally and internally, as their professional organisation.

## Association of Crossroads Care Attendant Schemes
10 Regent Place
Rugby
Warwickshire CV21 2PN
Tel: 01788 573653

For a care attendant to come and look after your relative at home.

## BACUP (British Association of Cancer United Patients)
3 Bath Place
Rivington Street
London EC2A 3JR
Tel:   0171-613 2121 (advice)
       0171-696 9003 (admin)
Freephone: 0800 181 199

Support and information for cancer sufferers and their families. Freephone advice line for people outside London.

## British Association of Domiciliary Care Officers (BADCO)
c/o Maggie Uttley
2 The Hornbeams
Swallowfield
Reading
Berkshire RG7 1QY
Tel: 01189 882954

## Carers National Association
20–25 Glasshouse Yard
London EC1A 4JS
Tel: 0171-490 8818 (admin)
Carersline: 0171-490 8898 (Mon–Fri, 1–4 pm)

Information and advice if you are caring for someone. Can put you in touch with other carers and carers' groups in your area.

## Citizens Advice Bureau

Listed in local telephone directories or in Yellow Pages under 'Social service and welfare organisations'. Other local advice centres may also be listed.

For advice on legal, financial and consumer matters. A good place to turn to if you don't know where to go for help or advice on any subject.

## Community Health Councils

Look in local telephone directory under the name of the Community Health Council where you live.

## Contact the Elderly
15 Henrietta Street
London WC2E 8QH
Tel: 0171-240 0630
Freephone helpline: 0800 716543
Fax: 0171-379 5781

Offers friendship to counter the loneliness of elderly people, particularly in their 80s and 90s, living alone.

## Counsel and Care
Lower Ground floor
Twyman House
16 Bonny Street
London NW1 9PG
Tel: 0171-485 1566

Advice for older people and their families; can sometimes give grants to help people remain at home, or return to their home.

## Cruse – Bereavement Care
126 Sheen Road
Richmond
Surrey TW9 1UR
Tel:  0181-940 4818/9047
     0181-332 7227 (bereavement line)
Fax: 0181-940 7638

Comfort in bereavement. Can put you in touch with people in your area.

## Disabled Living Foundation
380–384 Harrow Road
London W9 2HU
Tel: 0171-289 6111

Information about aids to help you cope with a disability.

## Help the Aged
16–18 St James' Walk
London EC1R 0BE
Tel: 0171-253 0253
Winter Warmth Hotline: 0800 289 404
Seniorline: 0800 650 065
Minicom: 0800 269626

Advice and information for older people and their families.

## Joint Initiative for Community Care Ltd
6 Minerva Gardens
Wavendon Gate
Milton Keynes MK7 7SR
Tel: 01908 585373

## Parkinson's Disease Society of the UK
72 Upper Woburn Place
London WC1H 0RA
Tel:  0171-383 3513
     0171-388 5798 (Helpline 10 am–4 pm)
Fax: 0171-383 5754

Information and advice for people caring for someone with Parkinson's disease; many local branches.

## Partially Sighted Society
PO Box 322
Doncaster DN1 2XA
Tel:   01302 368998
       0171-371 0289 (Helpline)

Advice and support for people with sight difficulties.

## Royal National Institute for Deaf People
19–23 Featherstone Street
London EC1Y 8SL
Tel: 0171-296 8000

Advice and support for people with hearing difficulties.

## Royal National Institute for the Blind
224 Great Portland Street
London W1N 6AA
Tel: 0171-388 1266

Advice and support for people with sight difficulties.

## Social Care Association
Thornton House
Hook Road
Surbiton
Surrey KT6 5AN
Tel: 0181-397 1411
Fax: 0181-397 1436

To promote and encourage a high standard of service for people receiving residential and day care.

## Standing Conference of Ethnic Minority Senior Citizens
5 Westminster Bridge Road
London SE1 7XW
Tel: 0171-928 7861

Information, support and advice for older people from ethnic minorities and their families.

## United Kingdom Home Care Association
42B Banstead Road
Carshalton Beeches
Surrey SM5 3NW
Tel: 0181-288 1551

Information about organisations providing home care in your area.


## LOCAL GOVERNMENT

### Local Government Association
26 Chapter Street
London SW1P 4ND
Tel: 0171-834 2222

### Local Government Management Board
Layden House
76–78 Turnmill Street
London EC1M 5QU
Tel: 0171-296 6600
Fax: 0171-296 6666


## TRADE UNIONS

### UNISON
1 Mabledon Place
London WC1H 9AJ
Tel: 0171-388 2366
Fax: 0171-387 6692

### UNISON EDUCATION
20 Grand Depot Road
London SE18 6SF
Tel: 0181-854 2244

# APPENDIX 9

# Further Reading

## COMMUNITY CARE – GENERAL

*Caring for People – Community Care in the Next Decade and Beyond*, Department of Health White Paper (HMSO, 1989).

*Department of Health Policy Guidance* (HMSO, 1990).

*Modernising Social Services*, Department of Health White Paper (The Stationery Office, 1998).

## HOME CARE

*Standards for Registration for Domiciliary Care*

*A Framework for the development of standards for delivering domiciliary care*

*Working with care: Health and safety in home care*

All developed by the Joint Advisory Group of Domiciliary Care Association. Available from the Social Care Association (Tel: 0181-397 1411).

*Taking Good Care: A handbook for care assistants* by Jenyth Worsley (Age Concern England, 1989).

## FINANCIAL MATTERS

Age Concern Factsheet 22, *Legal arrangements for managing financial affairs* (available free from Age Concern England at the address on p 242).

*Managing Other People's Money* by Penny Letts (Age Concern England, 1998).

## OTHER USEFUL PUBLICATIONS

*Community Life: A code of practice for community care* (1990) and *Home Life: A code of practice for residential care* (1984) [substantial overlap with issues relevant to home care provision]. Both available from Centre for Policy on Ageing, 25–31 Ironmonger Row, London EC1V 3PQ.

*Health and Healthy Living – A Guide for Older People* Department of Health (HMSO, 1991).

*Caring for Quality: An audit of the views of users of home care* (JICC, 1998). Available from JICC Ltd, 6 Minerva Gardens, Wavendon Gate, Milton Keynes MK7 7SR.

# APPENDIX 10

# Glossary

**Care awards** Those units which together make up one of the S/NVQs – the national qualifications in care. Each unit is sub-divided into elements and performance criteria (the standards).

**Care assessment** The process of identifying a person's need for care services.

**Care management** The process, which is carried out in various ways, of coordinating and arranging services for an individual person.

**Care manager** A person who carries out the major tasks of care management, such as assessment, preparing a care plan, coordinating services, and monitoring and review. The care manager may control the budget, but is not generally involved in providing a particular service.

**Care plan** The document which records the care needs, how the needs will be met and the required outcomes.

**Carer** A person who provides care and support for someone, but who is not employed to do so and is not part of the 'formal' sector (local and health authorities, voluntary organisations and the private sector).

**Community care** Services and support to help anyone with care needs to live as independently as possible in their home, wherever that is.

**Community care plans** Required annually of each local and health authority; to include information about the needs of the local population, and priorities and targets for meeting these, and to show how local authorities plan to stimulate the 'market' for care.

**Competence** The ability to undertake a task in practice or perform an activity to meet all the requirements of the national standard.

**Complaints procedure** The process which every social services department must have for listening and responding to comments and complaints from users (or potential users) of services.

**Contracting** The process through which local authorities purchase services from private or voluntary organisations.

**Eligibility criteria** Generally a level of care need which defines whether or not an individual is able to receive a service, and the urgency or priority of that need.

**Independent sector** Private, voluntary, charitable and not-for-profit organisations. For the purposes of spending the Special Transitional Grant, NHS trusts can be considered 'independent' of local authorities.

**Learning disability** Once described as 'mental handicap', or 'mental subnormality'. A permanent disability, usually occurring from birth, which affects learning abilities.

**Performance standards** The national standards against which competence is assessed (see also competence, care awards).

**Purchaser–provider split** The term sometimes used to describe the separation of two parts of one authority; one part assesses the needs of the local population and of individuals (the purchaser) and buys services from another part of the organisation (the provider). Also used to describe divisions of responsibility in the National Health Service.

**Respite care** Provides a break for a carer, either on a regular basis or occasionally. May be for just a few hours or for one or more weeks. May be provided in a person's own home or in a residential or nursing home or hospital.

**Risk assessment** An assessment of the personal physical risk involved in delivering the care service that is required.

**Statutory sector** Organisations created through Acts of Parliament – health authorities, local authorities, central government departments.

**Targeting** Identifying those in greatest need of services, and setting priorities to meet their needs.

**Value base** Those values which should underpin all practice in the provision of care.

# ABOUT AGE CONCERN

**Carefully** is one of a wide range of publications produced by Age Concern England, the National Council on Ageing. Age Concern cares about all older people and believes later life should be fulfilling and enjoyable. For too many this is impossible. As the leading charitable movement in the UK concerned with ageing and older people, Age Concern finds effective ways to change that situation.

Where possible, we enable older people to solve problems themselves, providing as much or as little support as they need. Our network of 1,400 local groups, supported by 250,000 volunteers, provides community-based services such as lunch clubs, day centres and home visiting.

Nationally, we take a lead role in campaigning, parliamentary work, policy analysis, research, specialist information and advice provision, and publishing. Innovative programmes promote healthier lifestyles and provide older people with opportunities to give the experience of a lifetime back to their communities.

Age Concern is dependent on donations, covenants and legacies.

**Age Concern England**
1268 London Road
London SW16 4ER
Tel: 0181-765 7200
Fax: 0181-765 7211

**Age Concern Cymru**
4th Floor
1 Cathedral Road
Cardiff CF1 9SD
Tel: 01222 371566
Fax: 01222 399562

**Age Concern Scotland**
113 Rose Street
Edinburgh EH2 3DT
Tel: 0131-220 3345
Fax: 0131-220 2779

**Age Concern Northern Ireland**
3 Lower Crescent
Belfast BT7 1NR
Tel: 01232 245729
Fax: 01232 235497

# PUBLICATIONS FROM AGE CONCERN BOOKS

## Care Professionals

### Working with Family Carers: A handbook for care professionals

Jacqui Wood with Phill Watson

Packed full of guidance and support, this multi-disciplinary handbook is designed to enable care professionals to view family carers as perhaps their greatest resource and to work in partnership with them. It provides clear and detailed information on every aspect of working with carers, both practically and emotionally. The authors – both experts in the field – offer practical tips and experience, on topics such as:

- financial difficulties
- emotional and physical stress
- relevant legislation
- ensuring carers' rights

Positive and supportive, this handbook will ensure that all front-line staff are fully armed in their fight to ensure carers receive the best possible support and help.

£14.99   0-86242-230-2

### Home Care: The Business of Caring

Linda How and Lesley Bell

Tackles head on, the problems faced by anyone either setting up or already running a home care business. Based on the experiences of purchasers and providers of home care, it is packed full of essential information and advice. Adopting an easy to follow question and answer format, this innovative publication will be an important resource to anyone who is thinking about setting up a home care business or anyone who already runs a business but still has questions to ask.

£14.99   0-86242-212-4

**Reminiscence and Recall: A guide to good practice (2nd Edition)**

Faith Gibson

This book aims to help carers become more competent in reaching out to older people in order to share their continuing journey towards growth, development and personal fulfilment. This new edition provides advice and guidance to develop and maintain the very highest standards in reminiscence work.

£11.99   0-86242-253-1

**Caring for Ethnic Minority Elders: A guide**

Yasmin Alibhai-Brown

A guide addressing the delivery of care to older people from ethnic minority groups, this book highlights the impact of varying cultural traditions and stresses their significance in the design of individual care packages. This book looks at the broader framework of how elders receive care and then considers the requirements and experiences of ten distinct ethnic minority groups.

. £14.99   0-86242-188-8

**The Community Care Handbook: The reformed system explained**

Barbara Meredith

Written by one of the country's leading experts, this hugely successful handbook provides a comprehensive overview of the implementation of the community care reforms and examines how the system has evolved.

£13.99   0-86242-171-3

# Money Matters

**Your Rights: A guide to money benefits for older people**

Sally West

A highly acclaimed guide to the State benefits available to older people. Contains information on Income Support, Housing Benefit and retirement pensions, among other matters, and provides advice on how to claim.

For further information, please telephone 0181-765 7200

**Managing Other People's Money (2nd Edition)**

Penny Letts

Foreword by the Master of the Court of Protection

The management of money and property is usually a personal and private matter. However, there may come a time when someone else has to take over on either a temporary or a permanent basis. This book looks at the circumstances in which such a need could arise and provides a step-by-step guide to the arrangements that have to be made.

£9.99    0-86242-250-7

---

If you would like to order any of these titles, please write to the address below, enclosing a cheque or money order for the appropriate amount made payable to Age Concern England. Credit card orders may be made on 0181-765 7200.

**Mail Order Unit**
Age Concern England
1268 London Road
London SW16 4ER

---

# INFORMATION LINE

Age Concern produces over 40 comprehensive factsheets designed to answer many of the questions older people – or those advising them – may have, on topics such as:

- finding and paying for residential and nursing home care
- money benefits
- finding help at home
- legal affairs
- making a Will
- help with heating
- raising income from your home
- transfer of assets

Age Concern offers a factsheet subscription service that presents all the factsheets in a folder, together with regular updates throughout the year. The first year's subscription currently costs £50; an annual renewal thereafter is £25. Single copies (up to a maximum of five) are available free on receipt of an sae.

---

To order your FREE factsheet list, phone 0800 00 99 66 (a free call) or write to:

**Age Concern**
FREEPOST (SWB 30375)
Ashburton
Devon TQ13 7ZZ

---

# INDEX